Wellness and Environmental Enrichment

Editor

AGNES E. RUPLEY

VETERINARY CLINICS OF NORTH AMERICA: EXOTIC ANIMAL PRACTICE

www.vetexotic.theclinics.com

Consulting Editor
AGNES E. RUPLEY

MAY 2015 • Volume 18 • Number 2

ELSEVIER

1600 John F. Kennedy Boulevard • Suite 1800 • Philadelphia, Pennsylvania, 19103-2899
http://www.vetexotic.theclinics.com

VETERINARY CLINICS OF NORTH AMERICA: EXOTIC ANIMAL PRACTICE Volume 18, Number 2
May 2015 ISSN 1094-9194, ISBN-13: 978-0-323-34187-5

Editor: Patrick Manley
Developmental Editor: Meredith Clinton

Veterinary Clinics of North America: Exotic Animal Practice (ISSN 1094-9194) is published in January, May, and September by Elsevier, Inc., 360 Park Avenue South, New York, NY 10010-1710. Subscription prices are $255.00 per year for US individuals, $399.00 per year for US institutions, $130.00 per year for US students and residents, $305.00 per year for Canadian individuals, $482.00 per year for Canadian institutions, $340.00 per year for international individuals, $482.00 per year for international institutions and $165.00 per year for Canadian and foreign students/ residents. To receive student/resident rate, orders must be accompanied by name of affiliated institution, date of term, and the *signature* of program/residency coordinator on institution letterhead. Orders will be billed at individual rate until proof of status is received. Foreign air speed delivery is included in all *Clinics* subscription prices. All prices are subject to change without notice. **POSTMASTER:** Send address changes to *Veterinary Clinics of North America: Exotic Animal Practice*, Elsevier Health Sciences Division, Subscription Customer Service, 3251 Riverport Lane, Maryland Heights, MO 63043. **Customer Service: Telephone: 1-800-654-2452** (U.S. and Canada); **1-314-447-8871** (outside U.S. and Canada). **Fax: 1-314-447-8029. E-mail: journalscustomerservice-usa@elsevier.com** (for print support); **journalsonlinesupport-usa@elsevier.com** (for online support).

Reprints. For copies of 100 or more of articles in this publication, please contact the Commercial Reprints Department, Elsevier Inc., 360 Park Avenue South, New York, New York 10010-1710. Tel.: 212-633-3874; Fax: 212-633-3820; E-mail: reprints@elsevier.com.

Veterinary Clinics of North America: Exotic Animal Practice is covered in *MEDLINE/PubMed (Index Medicus).*

Contributors

CONSULTING EDITOR

AGNES E. RUPLEY, DVM
Diplomate, American Board of Veterinary Practitioners (Avian Practice); Director and
Chief Veterinarian, All Pets Medical & Laser Surgical Center, College Station, Texas

EDITOR

AGNES E. RUPLEY, DVM
Diplomate, American Board of Veterinary Practitioners (Avian Practice); Director and
Chief Veterinarian, All Pets Medical & Laser Surgical Center, College Station, Texas

AUTHORS

MARTY McGEE BENNETT, BS
Founder, CAMELIDynamics, New Smyrna Beach, Florida

LEIGH ANN CLAYTON, DVM
Diplomate, American Board of Veterinary Practitioners (Avian and Reptile/Amphibian);
Director of Animal Health, Biological Programs Department, National Aquarium,
Baltimore, Maryland

MIKE CORCORAN, DVM, CertAqV
Associate Veterinarian, Arizona Exotic Animal Hospital, Mesa, Arizona; Founding Member,
American Association of Fish Veterinarians, Allentown, Pennsylvania; Certified Aquatic
Veterinarian, World Aquatic Veterinary Medical Association, Stafford, Staffordshire,
United Kingdom; VCA Wakefield Animal Hospital, Mesa, Arizona

LAUREL M. HARRIS, DVM
Wasatch Exotic Pet Care, Inc, Cottonwood Heights, Utah

MICHELLE G. HAWKINS, VMD
Diplomate, American Board of Veterinary Practitioners-Avian Practice; Associate
Professor, Avian and Exotic Medicine and Surgery, Department of Medicine and
Epidemiology, School of Veterinary Medicine, University of California-Davis, Davis, California

ANTHONY A. PILNY, DVM
Diplomate, American Board of Veterinary Practitioners (Avian); The Center for Avian and
Exotic Medicine, New York, New York

NANCI L.M. RICHARDS, DVM
Owner, Eastern Prairie Veterinary Service, St Joseph, Illinois

AGNES E. RUPLEY, DVM
Diplomate, American Board of Veterinary Practitioners (Avian Practice); Director and
Chief Veterinarian, All Pets Medical & Laser Surgical Center, College Station, Texas

ELISABETH SIMONE-FREILICHER, DVM
Diplomate, American Board of Veterinary Practitioners (AvianPractice); Senior clinician, Avian and Exotic Animal Medicine Department, MSPCA-Angell Animal Medical Center, Boston, Massachusetts

VALARIE V. TYNES, DVM
Diplomate, American College of Veterinary Behaviorists; Veterinary Services Specialist, CEVA Animal Health, Sweetwater, Texas

STACEY LEONATTI WILKINSON, DVM
Diplomate, American Board of Veterinary Practitioners (Reptile and Amphibian); Associate Veterinarian, Avian and Exotic Animal Care; Adjunct Assistant Professor, Department of Clinical Sciences, North Carolina State University College of Veterinary Medicine, Raleigh, North Carolina

Contents

Preface: Wellness Management and Environmental Enrichment of Exotic Pets   ix

Agnes E. Rupley

Keeping the Exotic Pet Mentally Healthy   187

Leigh Ann Clayton and Valarie V. Tynes

When basic needs are not met, captive animal health and welfare will be compromised by physical and psychological stressors. These basic needs include more than just appropriate food, water, and shelter; they should include environments that provide the animal with opportunities to thrive. These opportunities to thrive can be categorized as opportunity for a well-balanced diet (including how it is provided), to self-maintain, for optimal health, to express species-specific behaviors, and for choice and control. Adequate planning and knowledge are critical to creating environments in which animals can thrive.

Psittacine Wellness Management and Environmental Enrichment   197

Agnes E. Rupley and Elisabeth Simone-Freilicher

The goal of this article is to present practical ways to provide a healthier lifestyle to the commonly kept companion psittacine pets. Necessary information for bird owners to provide for the physical and mental health of their bird is presented. This information is exquisitely important for people keeping birds as pets to know and apply. It is the exotic veterinarian's responsibility to educate clients on how to provide properly for the pet's mental and physical well-being.

Juvenile Psittacine Environmental Enrichment   213

Elisabeth Simone-Freilicher and Agnes E. Rupley

Environmental enrichment is of great import to the emotional, intellectual, and physical development of the juvenile psittacine and their success in the human home environment. Five major types of enrichment include social, occupational, physical, sensory, and nutritional. Occupational enrichment includes exercise and psychological enrichment. Physical enrichment includes the cage and accessories and the external home environment. Sensory enrichment may be visual, auditory, tactile, olfactory, or taste oriented. Nutritional enrichment includes variations in appearance, type, and frequency of diet, and treats, novelty, and foraging. Two phases of the preadult period deserve special enrichment considerations: the development of autonomy and puberty.

Ferret Wellness Management and Environmental Enrichment   233

Laurel M. Harris

The domestic ferret is a commonly kept companion animal. Knowledge of proper husbandry of companion ferrets and their common disease processes by veterinarians assists pet owners in providing the healthiest environment possible. Attentiveness to the environmental needs of pet ferrets results in physically and psychologically healthy animals and a positive, enriched relationship with owners.

Small Exotic Companion Mammal Wellness Management and Environmental Enrichment   **245**

Anthony A. Pilny

Wellness management and environmental enrichment are important components of preventative veterinary medical care. Small exotic mammals represent a diverse group of pets with widely varying types of care, diet, and husbandry considerations; thus, environmental enrichment must go beyond the cage or tank design in order to provide proper mental fitness in meeting any pet's psychological needs. Addressing the pet's environmental, dietary, exercise, and social needs is vital to keeping these animals healthier and more disease resistant. The key to accomplishing this is largely impacted by the annual or biannual veterinary wellness visit and a commitment from the pet's owner.

Camelid Wellness   **255**

Marty McGee Bennett and Nanci L.M. Richards

Wellness management and environmental enrichment of New World camelids is multifaceted and should include everything from how they are fed and housed to how they are interacted with and handled. Camelid feeding regimens should be based on sound nutritional concepts, designed for specific animal groups, and begin with an appropriate forage base. Provide housing, shelter, substrate, and feeders designed for the needs and behaviors of camelids. Herd management should include regularly obtaining weights and body condition scores. Handling and training should be of a positive nature, in keeping with the natural history and temperament of the animal.

Reptile Wellness Management   **281**

Stacey Leonatti Wilkinson

Proper care and husbandry are the most important factors in keeping captive reptiles healthy. Improper nutrition, supplementation, caging, lighting, substrate, temperature, and humidity can all lead to stress and development of disease. Presented here are current recommendations for keeping captive reptiles. Care has moved away from sterile, spartan enclosures to larger, more naturalistic habitats. These habitats provide more space and choices for the reptile, leading to higher activity levels, reduced stress, and more opportunities to exhibit natural behaviors. Reptiles benefit from enrichment and are amenable to training in order to reduce stress and allow easier handling and veterinary care.

Environmental Enrichment for Aquatic Animals   **305**

Mike Corcoran

Aquatic animals are the most popular pets in the United States based on the number of owned pets. They are popular display animals and are increasingly used in research settings. Enrichment of captive animals is an important element of zoo and laboratory medicine. The importance of enrichment for aquatic animals has been slower in implementation. For a long time, there was debate over whether or not fish were able to experience pain or form long-term memories. As that debate has reduced and the consciousness of more aquatic animals is accepted, the need to discuss enrichment for these animals has increased.

Special Article

Advances in Exotic Mammal Clinical Therapeutics   323

Michelle G. Hawkins

It is important that veterinarians treating exotic companion mammals stay abreast of the latest developments relating to medications and drug delivery approaches for safety, efficacy and welfare issues. Sustained release formulations of commonly used drugs as well as newer routes for administration of therapeutic agents allow the veterinarian treating exotic companion mammals to reduce the stress associated with drug administration. Interactions can occur between vehicle and drugs when formulations are compounded, therefore research studies are warranted regarding potential problems associated with these formulations.

Index   339

VETERINARY CLINICS OF NORTH AMERICA: EXOTIC ANIMAL PRACTICE

FORTHCOMING ISSUES

September 2015
Endoscopy
Stephen J. Divers and Laila M. Proença,
Editors

January 2016
Soft Tissue Surgery
Kurt Sladky and Christoph Mans,
Editors

RECENT ISSUES

January 2015
Hematology
Terry Campbell, *Editor*

September 2014
Nutrition
Jörg Mayer, *Editor*

May 2014
Gastroenterology
Tracey K. Ritzman, *Editor*

RELATED INTEREST

Veterinary Clinics of North America: Small Animal Practice,
September 2013 (Vol. 43, No. 5)
Clinical Pharmacology and Therapeutics
Katrina L. Mealey, *Editor*

Preface

Wellness Management and Environmental Enrichment of Exotic Pets

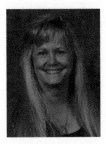

Agnes E. Rupley, DVM
Editor

This issue addresses the medical and physiologic needs of several species of exotic pets to help keep them healthy. It contains the information to provide quality care for exotic patients and to educate our clients on the care for their exotic pet's special needs: medical, environmental, and psychological.

This issue focuses on preventing and acquiring health and mental fitness rather than responding to illness after it has occurred. Such information will expand the exotic veterinarian's ability to provide total health care for exotic pets.

Presented are practical ways to provide a healthier lifestyle to our commonly kept companion exotic pets.

A health exam by a qualified veterinarian is a critical first step in any wellness plan; however, many exotic pet owners are seeking not only to provide for the medical health of their pet but also to become educated in providing for their pet's mental healthiness as well. Even if not sought by our clients, we as exotic pet veterinarians are the patient's advocates, and as such, we are obligated to provide our clients with the information to prevent disease and promote mental well-being. Effective approaches to provide exotic pets with sustainable help need to include understanding of the exotic pet's unique biology and behavior.

We can proactively educate owners about common health risks, prevention of behavior problems, and ways to promote health. We need to educate owners about needed lifestyle changes in reasonable and easily to implement strategies. These strategies include foraging and utilizing instinctive behavior to increase activity.

This issue is dedicated to those who enlightened us to the awareness of animal intelligence. God gave us dominion over the animals; however, with this comes the responsibility to care for the animal creatures He placed in our subjugation.

Vet Clin Exot Anim 18 (2015) ix–x
http://dx.doi.org/10.1016/j.cvex.2015.02.001
1094-9194/15/$ – see front matter © 2015 Published by Elsevier Inc.

vetexotic.theclinics.com

The goal of this issue is to create healthier, happier exotic pets. Educating the client on husbandry and behavior modification techniques unique to each species has the potential to improve the health and welfare of commonly kept exotic pets.

Agnes E. Rupley, DVM
All Pets Medical Center
111 Rock Prairie Road
College Station, TX 77845, USA

E-mail address:
agnesrupley@gmail.com

Keeping the Exotic Pet Mentally Healthy

Leigh Ann Clayton, DVM, DABVP (Avian and Reptile/Amphibian)[a],
Valarie V. Tynes, DVM, DACVB[b],*

KEYWORDS

- Welfare • Behavior • Behavioral health • Mental health
- Positive reinforcement training

KEY POINTS

- Chronic psychological stress can have a detrimental effect on the health and welfare of exotic pets.
- Environments that expose animals to aversive stimuli from which they cannot escape, unresolvable social conflict, unpredictable circumstances, or situations resulting in frustration or conflict can be highly stressful.
- Exotic pets should be given opportunities to thrive that include opportunity for a well-balanced diet, to self-maintain, to express normal species-specific behaviors, and to have choice and control over their environments.
- Exotic pet environments should also provide them with opportunities that decrease the likelihood that physical injury or disease will go unnoticed.

INTRODUCTION

Historically, there has been a tendency to separate physical (medical) and mental (behavioral) health conditions and treat them as if they were 2 separate entities. In this article, the term *mental health* encompasses behavioral and emotional health. With improving technology and growing medical knowledge, we are learning that physical and mental states are intricately interconnected, and there is not a sharp distinction between them. Physical health changes mental health and mental health can have profound effects on physical health, in the short and the long term. The veterinary clinician is equally responsible for both. This interconnection can be challenging for clinicians who have been trained to consider only the physical condition of their patients.

The authors have nothing to disclose.
[a] Biological Programs Department, National Aquarium, 501 East Pratt Street, 111 Market Place, Suite 800, Baltimore, MD 21202, USA; [b] CEVA Animal Health, PO Box 1413, Sweetwater, TX 79556, USA
* Corresponding author.
E-mail address: valarie.tynes@ceva.com

http://dx.doi.org/10.1016/j.cvex.2015.01.005
vetexotic.theclinics.com

The nonverbal status of veterinary patients is always a challenge, and both domesticated and wild species have evolved excellent mechanisms for masking signs of physical disease. Caretakers of exotic pets should educate themselves about the species' normal means of communication and practice studious observation of the animal's visual cues (body language) and behaviors. It is only by being familiar with normal behaviors of an animal that a caretaker is able to recognize the subtle changes that indicate declining welfare or impending illness. Veterinarians often gain experience recognizing and appreciating signs of physical disease during their careers. They may have less experience recognizing mental illness and psychological stress. Appreciating these states can be more challenging but extremely important to the well being of the exotic pet.

DOMESTICATED VERSUS WILD?

Caretakers of exotic animals must be acutely aware of the difference between a species that is fully domesticated verses one that is wild. Although species such as rabbits, hamsters, ferrets, and Guinea pigs are referred to as *exotic* pets, they have been domesticated. Because of artificial selection for traits desired by humans over many generations, individuals of these species are generally less fearful of people, more tolerant of novelty, and better able to adapt to captive environments. On the other hand, reptiles, most species in the order Psittaciformes, prairie dogs, and sugar gliders (among many others) are not domesticated and, although able to be tamed, individuals retain wild characteristics that can make adaptation to living with humans highly challenging. When individuals are unable to adapt to a given captive environment, the resulting psychological stress can lead to poor welfare. The species' status as predator or prey should also be taken into account. Prey animals, such as rodents, rabbits, and birds are likely to be stressed by the presence of predators and predator odors. This stress must be taken into account when housing multiple species in the same home. In addition, for many species, even domesticated ones, humans can be perceived as potential predators, and their presence can be highly stressful to some individuals. For this reason, one of the most important aspects caretakers of exotic pets can do is to take the time to habituate the animals to human presence. This habituation can be done with regular gentle handling if the animal seems to tolerate it well. Handling should always be associated with the offering of favored food, toys, play, or grooming, depending on what the animal perceives as reinforcing. Again, determining the best reinforcer takes careful practiced observation to recognize what the animal values. If the animal is extremely frightened of human presence, then simply dropping favored food items into the cage every time a person walks by can be enough to slowly habituate an animal to human presence and actually teach the animal to view the human as something pleasant to be anticipated.

STRESS AND MENTAL HEALTH

Stress has been defined in many ways, but for the purpose of this article, stress (or stressors) are defined as any physical, chemical, or emotional force that disturbs or threatens homeostasis, and the accompanying adaptive responses (the stress response) that attempt to restore homeostasis. The normal stress response is a result of the response of the sympathetic nervous system and the hypothalamic-pituitary-adrenal (HPA) axis. Within seconds of perceiving a stressor, the sympathetic nervous system secretes norepinephrine, and the adrenal medullae secretes epinephrine. This process prepares the body for a "fight or flight" response. The HPA axis is the body's primary physiologic stress response system.[1] When the HPA axis is triggered, the hypothalamus releases corticotrophin-releasing factor, which triggers the release of adrenocorticotropic hormone from the pituitary gland. The pituitary gland then stimulates the release of glucocorticoids from the adrenal cortex. Several other hormones, including prolactin, glucagon, thyroid hormones, and vasopressin, are secreted from other endocrine organs. The physiologic responses increase processes related to physical action and reduce processes not related to immediate survival. The overall effect of these 2 systems is to increase the immediate availability of energy, increase oxygen intake, decrease blood flow to areas not critical for movement, and inhibit digestion, growth, immune function, reproduction, and pain perception. In addition, memory and sensory function are enhanced. This system works well when responding to discrete short-term stresses.

However, if the system is chronically activated, the stress response persists and eventually becomes dysregulated. Chronic stress develops when an animal is unable to adapt to a particular stressor that does not go away (eg, the animal does not learn to cope with a particular aspect of its environment, does not habituate to certain frightening stimuli, or cannot escape an aversive environment). Cardiovascular, metabolic, reproductive, digestive, immune, and anabolic processes can be pathologically affected, subsequently leading to myopathy, fatigue, hypertension, decreased growth rates, gastrointestinal distress, suppressed immune function, and, ultimately, impaired disease resistance. Chronic stress leads to structural and functional changes in the brain, and, when extreme conditions persist, permanent damage can result.[2]

Chronic stress in animals can arise from both physical and psychological sources. Physical stressors include inappropriate food, temperature, humidity, substrate, or other basic environmental resources. Psychological stress may be a component of physical stressors (eg, not providing a climbing area for an arboreal species; **Box 1**) Chronic psychological stress can also arise from changing and unpredictable environments, social conflict, constant exposure to fear- or anxiety-provoking stimuli, and situations leading to frustration or conflict. Physically and psychologically stressful environments frequently occur when pet owners bring an animal into their home without having a complete understanding of its natural history and basic environmental and behavioral needs. Even more prepared caretakers may inadvertently cause psychological stress by misinterpreting behaviors associated with discomfort as a sign the animal likes something (eg, misinterpreting "freezing" in a rabbit as a sign that the animal finds human contact reinforcing). Wild species are more susceptible to chronic stress from fear-provoking stimuli associated with unpredictable environments and human encounters because of lack of selection for tolerance of humans and novelty.

There is certainly variation in how individuals perceive a given environmental stimulus or cope with the same environmental change. Thus, the same environment may cause a greater stress response in one animal compared with another. But, it is also well documented across species that psychological variables have a great deal of ability to modulate the stress response across individuals. These variables include control, predictability, and outlets for frustration (eg, displacement behavior). Being able to exert some control over a stressful situation is a coping mechanism; individuals that can control a situation causing them stress suffer fewer stress-related pathologies.[3] In a study in which one rat could control the rate of shocks received by pressing a lever, another rat received a shock every time the rat controlling the lever received a shock. Nevertheless, the rat that did not control the rate of shocks showed higher glucocorticoid concentrations than the rat with control of the shock.[4] Predictability also reduces the stress response. For example, rats receiving a warning signal before an electric shock had lower glucocorticoid concentrations than rats that did not

---

Box 1
Some important definitions

Conflict occurs when an individual is motivated to perform 2 opposing behaviors at the same time.

Frustration occurs when an individual is motivated to perform a particular behavior but is somehow prevented from doing so.

Displacement behavior is a normal behavior shown at an inappropriate time or out of context for the situation. Displacement behaviors often occur when an animal is experiencing conflict or frustration.

Fear is the emotion experienced when something is perceived as dangerous. Fear should result in the body preparing itself for appropriate action to avoid the fear-eliciting stimulus (fight or flight). Normally, fear should be an adaptive behavior allowing an animal to escape harm and live to reproduce its genetic material. However, animals can perceive danger when none is present, and, if unable to habituate, fear can become maladaptive. An animal existing in these circumstances would likely experience poor mental health and poor welfare. If the situation persisted without the animal learning to cope, the animal's subsequent stress response could be considered maladaptive and could ultimately lead to physical and or mental illness.

Anxiety is the anticipation of danger from unknown or imagined sources. The key word here is *imagined*. Caretakers must keep in mind that the danger is in the eye of the beholder. It is irrelevant if the danger is real or not; if the animal perceives something as threatening, it will respond with feelings of anxiety. The physiologic reaction is similar to that experienced when feeling fear and, in the long term, can be just as damaging.

Stress is any pressure or stress placed on a system or anything that threatens homeostasis. When the body's homeostasis is threated, the body's stress response system is activated in an attempt to regain homeostasis. If the animal is unable to respond either physiologically or behaviorally in a way that helps return its systems to homeostasis, then the stress response system may ultimately become dysregulated, leading to actual physical illness.

---

receive a warning signal.[5] The ability to engage in a displacement behavior has also been shown to ameliorate the effects of stress. Rats with access to a piece of wood to gnaw on during an electric shock also demonstrated relatively lower glucocorticoid concentrations compared with those that had no similar outlet.[5] Lastly, novelty, withholding of reward (or reinforcement), and the anticipation of punishment (not the punishment itself) have also been found to be potent psychological stressors.[2]

OPPORTUNITIES TO THRIVE

Creating environments that will enable animals to thrive and reduce or eliminate chronic stress is important for both the physical and mental health of exotic pets. Having a framework to help guide evaluation of an animal's environment that is applicable to any species is a useful tool for veterinarians and caretakers.

San Diego Zoo Global developed a 5-point animal welfare assessment guideline titled Opportunities to Thrive for internal use.[6] This program is derived from, and expands on, the commonly cited Five Freedoms created to evaluate farm animal welfare in the United Kingdom.[7] As opposed to The Five Freedoms, which largely guide caregivers on what to avoid, the 5 Opportunities to Thrive are action oriented and help guide caregivers on what to do to create environments that can work for animals.

The Opportunities to Thrive guidance serves as an exceptional framework that anyone working with animals, including exotic animal pets, can use to help support ongoing improvements in how animals are fed, housed, trained, and generally maintained. By continuously seeking to provide the optimum in animal caretaking, pet owners will at the same time be increasing the chance the pet will stay not only physically healthy but mentally and behaviorally healthy as well.

The opportunities to thrive are as follows:

1. Opportunity for a well-balanced diet—Fresh water and a suitable species-specific diet will be provided in a way that ensures full health and vigor, both behaviorally and physically.
2. Opportunity to self-maintain—An appropriate environment including shelter and species-specific substrates that encourage opportunities to self-maintain.
3. Opportunity for optimal health—Providing supportive environments that increase the likelihood of healthy individuals as well as rapid diagnosis and treatment of injury or disease.
4. Opportunity to express species-specific behavior—Quality spaces and appropriate social groupings will be provided that encourage species-specific behaviors at natural frequencies and of appropriate diversity while meeting social and developmental needs of each species in the collection.
5. Opportunities for choice and control—Providing conditions in which animals can exercise control and make choices to avoid suffering and distress and make behavior meaningful.

Opportunity for a Well-Balanced Diet

While providing for a well-balanced diet sounds like the most obvious of good husbandry guidelines, it is the latter part of the instruction that is typically overlooked by most pet owners—that the food be "provided in a way that ensures full health and vigor." In fact, how food is offered is equally important to an animal's health as what is offered. For example, wild psittacine birds spend most of their daily time budgets in search of food. Their natural behavioral repertoire includes much complex food acquiring and food manipulating behaviors. If all of their daily nutritional requirements, regardless of how well balanced, are provided in a single bowl, there is little else to occupy their day. It should come as no surprise that the animal is biologically incapable of filling its hours with very many other normal or appropriate behaviors. After all, thousands of years of evolution have gone into adapting its behaviors for the lifestyle it lives in the wild, not the lifestyle it lives in a cage. For this reason, caretakers of exotic pets should educate themselves about the natural history of the wild species they are acquiring, or the closest ancestor of a domestic species, so that they can, to the best extent possible, provide the animal with the nutritional needs in a manner that mimics how it would acquire food in the wild.

Opportunity to Self-Maintain

This requirement suggests that although good physical health may be maintained by providing an animal with the proper temperature, humidity, and substrate, at a bare minimum, good mental health also requires an animal be able to self-maintain by expressing its own comfort-seeking behaviors. These are the natural behaviors an animal would express in the wild, such as shade seeking when hot or shelter seeking when cold or in danger. For example, pigs seek out stationary objects in their environment to rub against, and some species of lizards seek flat rocks for basking. Caretakers will need to be aware of species' differences, for example, some species of reptiles prefer to burrow into substrate whereas others prefer a cavelike structure. Caretakers should be aware if the species they acquire is naturally nocturnal, diurnal, or crepuscular, as some nocturnal species will be highly stressed if given an environment in which they are unable to remove themselves from a bright active day time environment. A normal photoperiod is critically important for the good mental health of psittacines, and sleep deprivation is suspected to be a risk factor for many behavioral disorders in birds.[8]

Opportunity for Optimal Health

This opportunity can equally refer to supporting physical and mental health and the ability to rapidly identify and treat disease. Chronic, unrecognized, and untreated pain is found to be an important cause of anxiety and thus a stressor for all animals, including humans. If an animal exists in an environment in which injury or illness goes unrecognized, and thus untreated, the animal has the potential to suffer the mental health and poor welfare consequences of the process. In addition, unrecognized pain is often a cause for the sudden appearance of aggressive behaviors. The sudden onset of any behavioral change, especially aggression, in an adult animal, should always be followed by a complete physical examination and collection of a minimum database to rule out illness or injury.

Opportunities to Express Species-Specific Behavior

Providing animals the opportunity to engage in species-specific behavior is important at all stages of life, including the neonatal period. In this way, animals can develop more normal responses to future life events and learn normal social cues and interactions. This can be complicated when individuals are housed in situations in which fear of humans is learned or with parents who do not have normal social behaviors. Normal social groupings in the neonatal period may be particularly critical in avian species, notably psittacines, in which it is suspected that the early life stressors associated with premature separation from siblings and parents prevent them from developing normal social behavior and may predispose them to many problem behaviors.

It can take some forethought to develop environments that allow animals to express normal behaviors through all stages of their lives. Caretakers must be aware of whether the species they are acquiring is truly a species requiring social housing and the types of social groupings that are most appropriate. Providing appropriate social contact can be problematic. Social behaviors may involve antagonistic encounters and fairly sophisticated levels of understanding of the species' behavior may be needed to properly interpret interactions and ensure individuals are not put into chronically aversive or stressful settings. Some level of social disharmony may be appropriate and acceptable and part of the normal species' behavioral repertoire, but if it is too frequent or strong it can be a source of distress to some individuals. Human relations may provide some level of support for social needs in certain species, although with wild species, this is rarely enough for the development of normal behavioral patterns. For social species, housing in an appropriate grouping of conspecifics may be one of the most important aspects of their environment. For species that are normally solitary, housing them in social groups can be highly stressful and result in poor welfare.

Having adequate size and complexity of space (with enrichment that is biologically relevant for the species) is critical to ensuring species are able to express a broad range of normal behaviors. Caregivers should be encouraged to provide the largest possible housing for the animal. For example, most cages commercially available for pet rabbits and rodents are woefully undersized and not at all conducive to good mental or physical health for the animals. Understanding the natural history of the species is necessary to evaluate appropriateness of the enclosure shape and size and enrichment offered. For instance, the enclosure size, shape, and substrate will be different for a species that is arboreal compared with a fossorial species. In addition, the learning history of the individual should be taken into account. If an individual has had little exposure to enriched or novel environmental items, the caretaker must proceed at the animal's pace as enrichment opportunities are expanded.

Opportunities for Choice and Control

It is now generally accepted that the ability to exercise choice and control is fundamental to good welfare and health in animals (including humans). Multiple studies across genuses have found similar positive behavioral and physiologic responses to environments rich in choice and control and found negative impacts when opportunities for choice and control are limited.

The environment should provide opportunities to engage in a variety of behaviors that can gain positive reinforcement and support a large behavioral repertoire. In addition, the animal can make a choice to not perform a given behavior (eg, it can choose to build a nest from cotton but not shavings). A choice to not perform a behavior should carry no adverse effect, particularly when interacting with caregivers (eg, if the animal chooses to not come toward the caretaker but instead moves away, the caretaker allows the animal to move away rather than picking up the animal). Broadly speaking, creating environments that are rich in opportunities to gain positive reinforcement are recommended. This can be done by providing a highly enriched environment and engaging in deliberate training programs based on positive reinforcement. Examples of enrichment include giving the animal access to various areas, substrates, temperatures, foods, foraging opportunities, and training sessions that are based on positive reinforcement. Good welfare is created when individual animals can choose what to do to gain positive reinforcement and are free to use behavior to escape aversive situations. The general balance of interactions with the environment is such that there is a strong shift toward positive reinforcement.

The use of deliberate positive reinforcement training for wild animals under professional care has increased markedly across taxa in the recent decades. Positive reinforcement training allows animals to participate willingly in their care (eg, offer body parts for examination, venipuncture, and wound treatment). Animals also learn they have choice in whether to interact with human caretakers, and this is proving to be extremely beneficial to their well-being.[9] One recent study found that this type of formal training significantly reduced fear of humans, which in the long term would benefit welfare.[10] There is no reason to think that this type of training would not be equally beneficial to all exotic pets.

Introducing some basic positive reinforcement training will increase the amount of positive reinforcement in the environment. Because many of these terms are often used in a confusing manner, **Box 2** and **Table 1** are included to clarify the definitions

---

Box 2
Important definitions for understanding how animals learn

Reinforcement is any stimulus that increases the likelihood of a behavior being repeated.

Positive reinforcement involves the presentation of something that is likely to strengthen a behavior response. (It increases the likelihood that the behavior will be repeated.) This will need to be something of value to the individual. Food is often the most valuable reinforcer for animals simply because it is necessary for life.

Negative reinforcement involves the removal of something unpleasant that strengthens the behavior response. A common example is an animal biting a human hand to get the hand to go away.

Punishment is any stimulus that decreases the likelihood of a behavior being repeated.

Positive punishment involves the application of something unpleasant or aversive, such as a shock, verbal reprimand, squirting with water, or threatening with a newspaper.

Negative punishment involves the removal of something pleasant, such as play, the potential for food rewards, or social interaction.

Table 1		
Consequences and functions involved in operant learning		
	Function	
Operation	**Increase the Behavior**	**Decrease the Behavior**
Addition +	Positive reinforcement (rewards)	Positive punishment (discipline)
Subtraction −	Negative reinforcement (escape from something unpleasant)	Negative punishment (Loss of something desirable)

of positive reinforcement. The definition of the term and how it differs from negative reinforcement and punishment are also explained. This can serve to improve the relationship between the animal and the caretaker and build trust. Targeting (having the animal touch a part of its body—usually the nose—to a target) is a commonly recommended foundation behavior. Targeting is usually easily trained and can be trained in a protected contact situation (animal in the regular enclosure with the person outside of the enclosure) to help ensure the person is not inadvertently using force when training the behavior. Food reinforcement can be deposited in front of or near the animal so that the animal is not required to approach the person and take food directly from his or her hand, an act that can lead to a great deal of mental conflict for many animals. This type of training can be especially important if working with fearful animals, such as a bird that has had limited human interaction. Target training can be accomplished with any exotic pet.

For many humans, our "cultural inheritance" is that animals should do what we say just because we ask for it. There is even widespread fear that providing positive reinforcement for desired behavior will create spoiled animals. However, the science of behavior analysis (the study of how individuals learn) tells us that the way to increase or sustain behavior is to ensure that the behavior is positively reinforced. If there is not positive reinforcement associated with behavior, the behavior will not be maintained. Behavior is costly in terms of time and energy. Repeating behaviors that are not reinforced does not make biological sense. Learning the basics of behavior analysis and the skills for using positive reinforcement training techniques allows veterinarians to better guide caregivers in the appropriate use with exotic pets.

It takes effort and thought to control our interactions with animals and to move toward providing greater choice and control. It will not happen randomly. Veterinarians can help improve the physical and mental health of exotic pets by encouraging owners to create environments rich in opportunities for positive reinforcement by providing foraging, positive reinforcement training, and variety that works for the individual and species. Caregivers should also be supported in reducing their unintentional use of forceful methods of controlling animals. Many exotic pets are physically small; it is easy to pick them up and move them, ignoring body language that indicates the animal is not comfortable.

SUMMARY

Captive animals often have their behavior significantly constrained, including exotic pets. Major events in their lives are dictated by the schedule of the human caregiver—when food is delivered, how food is presented, how they are interacted with, control of their movements, exposure to temperature extremes, ability to respond to environmental changes, physical contact, and exposure to conspecifics. Their behavior repertoire is much smaller than a wild counterpart, and this constraint of their behavioral repertoire is theorized to be a root cause of many common behavioral problems. At the least, it is likely to stress the animal, contribute to poor mental health, predispose them to physical illness, and ultimately result in poor welfare. Veterinarians can play an integral role in improving the welfare of captive exotic pets by being informed about the role of stress in mental and physical health and the importance of providing animals with environments with choices, control, and multiple opportunities for expressing a variety of normal behavior patterns.

REFERENCES

1. Hennessy MB. Using hypothalamic–pituitary–adrenal measures for assessing and reducing the stress of dogs in shelters: a review. Appl Anim Behav Sci 2013;149(1–4):1–12.
2. McEwen BS. The neurobiology of stress: from serendipity to clinical relevance. Brain Res 2000;886:172–89.
3. Gatchel RJ, Baum A, Krantz DS. An introduction to health psychology. 2nd edition. New York: Newberry; 1989.
4. Weiss JM. Effects of coping response on stress. J Comp Physiol Psychol 1968; 65:251–60.
5. Sapolsky RM. Neuroendocrinology of the stress response. In: Becker JB, Breedlove SM, Crew D, editors. Behavioral endocrinology. Cambridge (MA): MIT Press; 1992. p. 287–324.
6. Janssen DL, Miller L, Vicino G. Animal welfare and behavior: opportunities to thrive. 46th AAZV Annual Conference. Orlando (FL), October 18–24, 2014.
7. Farm Animal Welfare Committee, Department of Environment, Food, and Rural Affairs, United Kingdom. Five Freedoms. Available at: http://www.defra.gov.uk/fawc/about/five-freedoms/. Accessed February 19, 2015.
8. Seibert LM, Sung W. Psittacines. In: Tynes VV, editor. The behavior of exotic pets. Oxford (United Kingdom): Wiley-Blackwell; 2010. p. 1–11.
9. Heidenreich B. An introduction to the application of science-based training technology. Vet Clin North Am Exot Anim Pract 2012;15:371–85.
10. Ward SJ, Melfi V. The implications of husbandry training on zoo animal response rates. Appl Anim Behav Sci 2013;147:179–85.

Psittacine Wellness Management and Environmental Enrichment

Agnes E. Rupley, DVM, DABVP (Avian)[a],*,
Elisabeth Simone-Freilicher, DVM, DABVP (Avian Practice)[b]

KEYWORDS

- Psittacine • Wellness care • Environmental enrichment • Foraging • Pet birds

KEY POINTS

- Client education is critical to the physical and mental well-being of the pet psittacine bird.
- Appropriate nutrition and diet conversion are keys to good physical health.
- The goals of environmental enrichment are to increase activity and promote a wide diversity of natural behaviors.
- Physical environmental enrichment helps to alleviate boredom by giving birds more activity choices.
- The welfare of the pet bird depends on the knowledge and motivation of the owner. Much is required to provide suitable mental and physical caretaking.

There are multiple challenges in keeping mentally and physically healthy psittacine birds as pets. Significant aspects of natural parrot behavior are denied to varying degrees for parrots kept as companion animals. Examples of these include flocking, social interaction with other birds, foraging on a variety of foods, and flight. Birds are social, loud, and messy. When kept in captivity, they deserve the owners' tolerance to exhibit these normal behaviors.

Many psittacine birds are long-lived and deserve continuity of quality care by familiar diligent caregivers. Their social interaction needs are demanding. Their intelligence requires intellectual stimulation. Inadequate care is an extremely important welfare issue and can have detrimental mental and health consequences. Pet birds should be provided with social companionship. Owners are often the only social interaction for a pet bird and must serve the functions of the flock. Examples include answering contact calls, playing,

The authors have no affiliation with any product or service mentioned in this article.
[a] All Pets Medical Center, 111 Rock Prairie Road, College Station, TX 77845, USA;
[b] MSPCA-Angell Animal Medical Center, 350 South Huntington Avenue, Boston, MA 02130, USA
* Corresponding author.
E-mail address: agnesrupley@gmail.com

preening, and talking with the bird. Opportunities should be provided to involve the bird in family activities.

Welfare may be improved by appropriate environmental enrichment and changes in the social environment; however, such changes require that caretakers have sufficient motivation, knowledge, and resources to provide these essential necessities. When these requirements are not met, the bird experiences mental and physical suffering.

Veterinarians who treat birds have an obligation to be the pet's advocate. Bird-owning clients must be educated about crucial physical and mental needs of their special companions. Although exceptions exist and requirements vary among species, keeping birds as pets has resulted in serious welfare issues for these challenging pets. Birds may be unsuitable as human companions.[1]

All pets deserve the following 5 freedoms[2]:

1. Freedom from hunger and thirst (access to a healthy diet and clean water)
2. Freedom from discomfort (appropriate environment, including shelter and comfortable resting area)
3. Freedom from pain, injury, and disease (prevention or rapid diagnosis and treatment)
4. Freedom to express normal behavior (sufficient space, suitable environment, and social interaction)
5. Freedom from fear and distress (conditions and treatment that avoid mental suffering) (**Box 1**).

HUSBANDRY
Nutrition

There is a plethora of information on diets for pet birds, and knowledge of the best nutrition continues to develop. Birds need a proper balance of carbohydrates, proteins, fats, vitamins, minerals, and water. Detailed nutritional information is beyond the scope of this article. For further information on psittacine nutrition, consult "Clinical Avian Nutrition" by S. Orosz[3] and other resources.

Nutrition and enrichment are frequently neglected essentials of most pet bird owners. Often owners mistakenly believe they are providing suitable nutrition. Inadequate nutrition is a common source of health problems. It is not sufficient to feed birds what they need just to keep them alive; instead, they must be provided such that they flourish. Their health will be contingent on nutrition and enrichment.

Box 1
Tips for keeping pet birds happy

- Choose an appropriate species based on noise level, space requirements, and intelligence.
- When possible, choose a parent-weaned bird rather than a hand-weaned or unweaned bird.
- Follow a daily routine, providing meals, attention, and activities in a predictable order.
- Provide foraging opportunities.
- Use positive reinforcement for training.
- Provide a quiet area for a minimum of 10 to 12 hours of uninterrupted sleep each night.
- Provide daily opportunities for exercise (eg, flapping, running, swinging, flight).
- Regularly rotate or offer a variety of nontoxic, bird-safe toys.

Adapted from Seibert LM. Husbandry considerations for better behavioral health in psittacine species. Compendium 2007;1–4.

Physical and mental health of pet birds requires that proper nutrition and environmental needs be taught to the owner. Psittacines in the wild and in captivity do not consistently select foodstuffs that are nutritionally adequate.[4] Owners often provide a variety of foodstuffs falsely thinking the bird will self-balance its diet, believing they are providing good nutrition. However, this assumption is incorrect. In addition, rich foods may not only provide inadequate nutrition but also contribute to obesity and abnormal reproductive behaviors.

Nutritionally complete diets developed and tested through feeding trials are recommended for at least 50% to 80% of the *consumed* calories. Appropriate vegetables, fruits, grains, and high protein foodstuffs can compose approximately 20% to 50% of the diet, partially depending on species of bird. Natural berries and dark green, red, and orange vegetables and fruits generally have a high nutrient content and are recommended. Cooked meat, fish, eggs, rice, grains, and pieces of nuts also can be offered. Pale vegetables, with a high water composition (iceberg or head lettuce, celery), offer little nutritional value. Preparation of fruits and vegetables requires that they be washed well to remove bacteria, insecticides, and other chemicals. Avoid feeding foods with high fat and sugar content, chocolate, caffeine, alcohol, and possibly, avocados. It is recommended that peanuts be avoided because of the potential presence of aflatoxins, which can cause liver failure. Inform clients to provide a few selections each day, but to vary the selections between days. They should continue to offer a variety of foods, because preferences change over time (**Table 1**).

Research and feeding trials have been used to help determine the ideal content of many available formulated diets. The feeding of these diets has improved the health of pet psittacine birds; however, diet conversion, lack of variety and lack of opportunity for birds to display innate foraging behavior are problems that need to be addressed. Converting a bird to a formulated diet is not always easy. Birds may not recognize new foodstuffs as food. Diet conversion should be attempted only in healthy birds. A variety of strategies can be used to aid in converting birds to formulated diets (**Box 2**).

Table 1
Some suggested nutritious vegetables and fruits

Apricots	Asparagus
Blackberries	Broccoli
Brussels sprouts	Cantaloupe
Carrots and carrot tops	Cherries
Corn (fresh, on the cob, canned)	Figs
Kale	Kiwi
Lettuce (leaf)	Mangos
Melons	Nectarines
Oranges	Papaya
Peas	Peppers (red/yellow/green/fresh/dried)
Peaches	Pomegranate
Pumpkin	Raspberries
Spinach	Squash
Strawberries	Sweet potatoes
Swiss chard	Tangerines
Tomatoes	

Avoid dried fruits; these have a high sugar content.

Box 2
Diet conversion strategies

- Use natural behavior characteristics as effective tools for diet conversion, including their highly visual character, innate curiosity, feeding habits, and enjoyment of drama.

- Let the bird see the owner examining and appearing to eat the new food. The owner can pick up the new food and with great drama show interest in relishing these pieces of new food, then offering a portion to their bird. It may take several sessions for the bird to try these new foods.

- Allow the bird to eat with the owner, offering new foodstuffs. Do not offer food that has come in contact with a human mouth because of the human normal oral bacterial flora.

- Sprinkle familiar food mixed with some of the new diet on a table, then act enthusiastic as the bird shows interest in the new foods.

- Skewer foods and attach in the cage near a favored perch.

- Birds are often wary of new items placed in their cages. Place new foods in the currently used food bowls in their familiar locations.

- Prime eating time is when the bird first wakes up. Birds tend to eat vigorously at sunrise. Sunrise may be outside light filtering through windows, uncovering of the cage, or a light switched on. Having the new food in the cage at this time increases the likelihood for exploration of the new food.

- Place the new food in the regular food bowl. Allow access to the regular diet twice daily for 15 minutes. Have the new food in the cage at sunrise. Do not allow the bird to lose more than 10% of its body weight using this strategy. It can take weeks to months for diet conversion; however, consistency and persistence are often required.

Weight Management

Weight management is often needed because of the diet fed and inactivity of pet psittacine birds. Ideally, birds would be able to fly and exercise daily in a safe environment. Foraging, teaching and performing tricks, and toys are other ways to increase activity. Feeding a nutritious diet with an appropriate fat content based on the species of bird is recommended (see Nutrition above).

Water

Clean pathogen-free water should be provided at all times. Water bowls and perches should be placed such that droppings do not contaminate the water. Water bowls should be washed daily with soap and water. They should be allowed to dry completely before use. Sipper water bottles are not recommended unless cleaned daily with soap and water and allowed to dry completely before use. Many birds will bathe if a large bowl of water is provided for this behavior. In addition, many birds also enjoy daily misting with a spray bottle from above.

Housing

The cage should be made from nontoxic material with appropriately spaced bars. Ideally, it would be large enough for flight. If this is not possible, the largest cage the owner can afford and has the space for is recommended. Minimum size required is adequate space for the bird to spread its wings without hitting either the sides of the cage or other perches; room to forage, climb, balance, walk, and play; and adequate space for multiple perches, toys, and food and water bowls. A variety of perch sizes, and possibly variety of textures, should be provided. Sandpaper-covered perches are hazardous and therefore should not be used. Time outside the cage for birds to experience normal behaviors of flight and social interaction is a necessity.

A place should be provided in the cage where the bird feels safe and can retreat when wanted. Depending on the species and temperament, birds generally benefit from a certain amount of commotion and may become vocal and playfully excited by sounds. Normal activities of the human flock about the house, television, vacuum cleaner, an electric razor, cooking, and music and recordings of other birds and sounds of nature are examples of potentially exciting sounds. Excessively loud noises and even normal activity may cause undue stress for some birds. Remember the bird is captive in its environment and cannot freely escape these sounds and activities. Exposure to noise should be limited to the bird's normal waking hours.

Dust, fecal matter, bits of food, dirt, and feather dust accumulate constantly on the cage and everything in it. The entire cage should be cleaned at least once weekly. Food and water bowls must be positioned to prevent contamination with droppings. As noted earlier, food and water bowls should be cleaned daily with soap and water and then allowed to dry before reusing.

Cage Substrate

Cage bottoms and enclosure floors must be kept clean. Disposable paper lining such as newspaper or paper towels, discarded daily, allows for daily inspection of the droppings. Ideally, bars prevent the bird's access to older food and droppings. Several layers of paper can be placed at the bottom of the cage, removing one layer daily, which allows for evaluation of droppings. Although not usually specific for any one particular disease, a change in the color, frequency, volume, or character of droppings indicates a health problem that requires immediate attention. Polyuria, increased fluid in the dropping, is often the first symptom of illness in birds. The amount of feces indicates food intake or passage through the digestive tract. It is recommended that the newspaper be separated from the bird by bars to prevent nesting behaviors and ingestion of old and fecal-contaminated foods.

Some substrates can cause health problems. Wood shavings can cause respiratory problems. Corncob bedding can contain fungal spores, and if a bird is able to reach the corncob substrate, it can be ingested and cause impaction. Corncob bedding also retains moisture from the droppings and spilled water, providing a prime breeding ground for bacteria and mold. The bacteria and mold can be inhaled and cause infections. Also, droppings cannot be accurately evaluated daily in corncob and shavings.

Lighting

Sleep and reproductive behaviors are affected by the quality and length of uninterrupted darkness. A dark quiet sleeping area is recommended.

The type of artificial lighting should be carefully considered. Birds see light from fluorescent light bulbs as blinking like a strobe light. Critical flicker fusion frequency is the minimal number of flashes of light per second at which an intermittent light stimulus no longer stimulates a continuous visual sensation. Light from fluorescent bulbs appears constant to humans; however, these bulbs emit light discontinuously. Their flickering is invisible to most humans under normal conditions, but might be detectable by some species of birds.[5] Incandescent or LED lights are recommended. For more information on flicker fusion frequency, see the article entitled, "Behavioral Assessment of Flicker Fusion Frequency in Chicken Gallus gallus domesticus" by Thomas J. Lisney.[5]

ENVIRONMENTAL ENRICHMENT
What Is Environmental Enrichment?

Environmental enrichment describes improved living conditions. It is the process of enhancing the pet's environment using its behavioral biology and natural environment characteristics. It is providing opportunities for birds to hide, socialize, exercise, and occupy time. Environmental enrichment increases the bird's behavior choices, draws out their species-appropriate behaviors, and enhances their mental welfare. Environmental enrichment plans should be holistic, involving all aspects of the environment. Realistically, it means shifting from a very impoverished environment to a less impoverished environment (**Boxes 3** and **4**).

Why Is Environmental Enrichment Important?

Psittacine birds are intelligent creatures. Keeping such intelligent animals in captivity and in artificial environments can induce suffering, unwanted negative behaviors, and stereotypes. Stereotypical behaviors include aggression, feather damaging and picking, self-mutilation, excessive fearfulness, and abnormal repetitive, unvarying, and functionless behaviors. These behaviors are the result of not allowing the bird the opportunities to express natural behaviors or exercise normally. Animals housed in artificial habitats may experience environmental challenges that result in stress, adversely affecting them.[6] Some sources of stress include artificial lighting, exposure to loud or aversive sounds, restricted movement, reduced or lack of retreat space, forced proximity to humans, and reduced feeding opportunities. Psittacine birds are social animals that interact with their flock. When kept as pets, they often lack the critically important interaction that provides for their mental well-being.

Physical environmental enrichment helps to alleviate boredom by giving them more activity choices. It encourages them to search for, explore, and manipulate their food in ways more normal to their natural biology. Foraging for food, play, and exploration are some of the activities that can mentally stimulate them and help prevent boredom. Preventing boredom helps to avert abnormal behavior and stereotypic behaviors.

Box 3
Ten behavior categories identified in a study of birds' activity in the wild

1. Foraging: reaching for, manipulating, and ingesting food items

2. Resting: perching

3. Resting alert: perching with some body movement

4. Maintenance behavior: auto-preening, bill wiping, scratching, shaking, stretching, and bathing

5. Climbing or walking

6. Flying

7. Billing: use of beak without associated feeding

8. Aggressive behavior: chasing and fighting

9. Reproductive behavior: including nest formation and maintenance

10. Vocalizing

Categories are not mutually exclusive.
Adapted from Bauck L. Psittacine diets and behavioral enrichment. Semin Avian Exotic Pet Med 1998;7(3):135–40; with permission.

Box 4
Five categories of enrichment

1. Social enrichment includes interaction with conspecifics, interaction with other animals, interaction with people, and interaction with other (mirror, look-alike, plush toy).

2. Cognitive enrichment includes mental stimulation (puzzle feeders, training session) and the novel experiences (unusual food, novel item, unusual scent).

3. Physical habitat enrichment includes perching/climbing structures (texture, diameter, motion, resting spots), substrates, protected area (from people, animals, elevation, viewpoint, partial visual barrier), and climate (light, temperature, humidity, wind).

4. Sensory enrichment includes tactile, olfactory and taste, auditory (vocalizations, "white" noise, noise makers, videos, music), and visual. Birds have sensory abilities far beyond human capabilities in the range of vision spectrum and hearing.

5. Food enrichment includes novel food items and food presentation (puzzle feeders, multiple food bowls, hidden food).

Initiation of environmental enrichment is beneficial at any stage of a bird's life.
Adapted from The Shape of Enrichment Inc. Available at: http://www.enrichment.org/. Accessed February 16, 2015; and CCAC training module on: environmental enrichment, Canadian Council on Animal Care. Available at: http://www.ccac.ca/en_/training/niaut/vivaria/enrichment. Accessed February 16, 2015.

It is the responsibility of veterinarians who treat these pets to educate clients such that they can provide for the optimal well-being of the pets entrusted to their care.

How Is Environmental Enrichment Provided?

Providing opportunities to occupy bird's waking hours that simulate normal habits and behaviors promote mental health. Foraging for food, play, and exploration are some of the activities that can help pass time and prevent boredom. The goal of environmental enrichment is to increase activity and promote a wide diversity of natural behaviors. Environmental enrichment is accomplished through stimulating investigation and interaction with surroundings by presenting novel objects and toys, objects, and/or perches on which to chew; periodic rearranging the structures in the cage; and intermittent changing of the places and ways foods are presented. Birds often enjoy swings (**Fig. 1**).

Birds may have to be taught how to live as a bird in the confines of the human social structure of its environment. Environmental enrichment will not be beneficial if the environmental modification has little functional significance to the animal.[7] Birds can be taught by observation of a human or another bird in their environment to actively engage and enjoy interacting with toys and their environment as well as seek and find food.

One of the favorite pastimes of psittacine birds is to make little things out of big things. Natural wood perches, perches with bark, wooden toys, shredders (**Fig. 2**), and any nontoxic safe material can be offered. For birds fearful of novel items, slow introduction through wrapping the toy or gradually moving the toy closer to the cage is recommended.

Environmental enrichment can also be provided with water. Daily misting using a spray bottle can be offered. Most birds prefer the mist to fall from above rather than direct spraying. Some birds prefer water dishes in which to bathe either in or out of

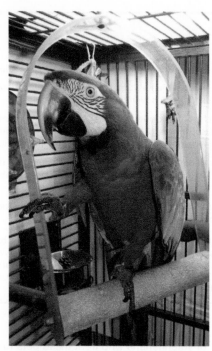

Fig. 1. Swings provide excellent exercise and balancing effort.

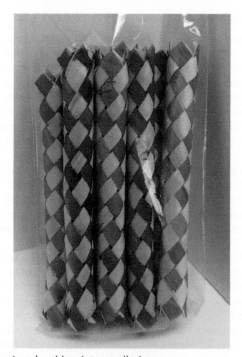

Fig. 2. Birds enjoy tearing shredders into small pieces.

the cage. Showering with owners, having a perch within the shower to rest on, is enjoyed by many birds. Bathing and misting also encourage normal preening behavior.

The presence of a normal range of behaviors and the absence of abnormal behaviors or stereotypic behaviors are indicators of providing adequate environmental enrichment.

Foraging

In the wild, psittacine birds spend considerable time foraging for food; for example, glossy cockatoos were found to spend 88% of the day engaged in feeding activities.[8] Foraging is a way to increase the time spent seeking and eating food (**Fig. 3**).

Foraging behaviors often must be taught to birds. Foraging can be done inside and outside the cage. Novelty enrichment can be achieved by providing food with different colors, textures, sizes, and smells. Pelleted food, vegetables, fruits, pieces of nuts, whole nuts (if species appropriate), treats, and Nutriberries can be used for foraging (**Box 5, Fig. 4**).

Acceptance of new foods is often quickly explored when added to a skewer (**Fig. 5**).

Providing owners with the information needed to provide foraging will increase the likelihood of meeting this important basic need. Captive Foraging DVD by Dr Scott Echols[9] is an excellent resource on foraging for clients.

Exercise

Exploratory behavior is an important component of a normal bird's daily routine (**Fig. 6**).

Physical enrichment can include toys, swings, ladders, mirrors, and providing a large flying room. Toys are an important part of a bird's life. Toys of the appropriate size for the bird are recommended. Appropriate toys can be made of wood, acrylic, rawhide, or rope (**Figs. 7–9**).

There are hanging toys, foot toys, puzzle toys, and those that attach to the side of the cage. A variety of toys are recommended. Toys come in varying difficulty (**Fig. 10**).

Toys can be bought or made (**Fig. 11**).

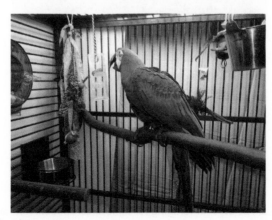

Fig. 3. Foraging inside a cage.

Box 5
Foraging ideas

Insert food in toys

Skewer food

Hide food in crushed paper bags, newspaper, small paper plates, coffee filters, Dixie cups, corn husks, or snow-cone cups and wedge between the cage bars

Put food in multiple food bowls in different areas of the cage

Cover food bowls with paper, cardboard, or wood

Mix food among toys or other inedible items

Wedge pieces of nuts and treats into holes of wooden and plastic toys, then hang from the cage or toys

Hide food or treats among toys, shredded paper, or other inedible items

Weave greens in cage bars

Hide food in cardboard boxes

Purchase foraging toys, as many are available

Create foraging containers be easily at home; however, ensure materials used are safe

---

Rotating toys weekly is recommended to maintain interest. Some species and some birds may prefer natural enrichment items, such as foods and branches, rather than nonnatural toys (**Fig. 12**).

Birds occasionally must be taught how to play and how to explore their environment.

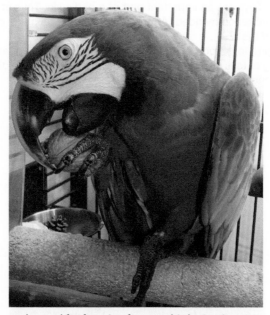

Fig. 4. Whole nuts can be used for foraging for some birds. Caution: Nuts are high in fat and calories.

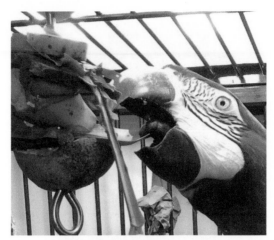

Fig. 5. Acceptance of new foods are often quickly explored when added to a skewer.

HEALTHY OWNER AND BIRD INTERACTION

Learning by both the owners and the bird is always occurring. Teaching owners how to use positive reinforcement to train and to build desirable behaviors is an essential learning. Positive reinforcement and respect for the bird's wanting or not wanting interaction and rewards should be respected at all times. Owners of pet birds should treat them in a manner that minimizes discomfort and stress.

Training commands, tricks, and flying will benefit the bird mentally and physically. A perch shaped like a T is an excellent training resource. While the bird is perched

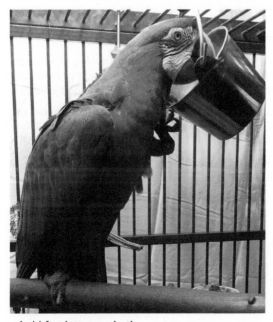

Fig. 6. A bucket can hold food, toys, or both.

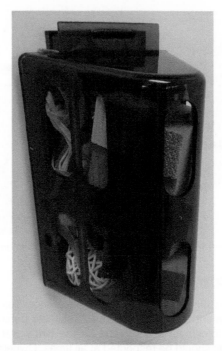

Fig. 7. Bright-colored acrylic toy containing smaller beak and foot toys.

on the T, the teaching of tricks and the giving of commands can occur. This training provides exercise, mental stimulation, and positive reinforcement based on the owner's reaction. An important job of the avian veterinarian is teaching owners to use positive reinforcement with their bird to build their relationship and promote desirable behaviors.

Some bird training Web sites include the following:

- Barbara Heidenreich's Force Free Animal Training at: www.BarbarasFFAT.com
- Parrot Training at: www.GoodBirdInc.com and http://www.goodbirdinc.com/
- Lafeber at: http://lafeber.com/pet-birds/avian-expert-articles/

Exercise serves as a means to reduce or eliminate unwanted behaviors. For every established behavior the owner wishes to reduce or eliminate, time needs to be spent

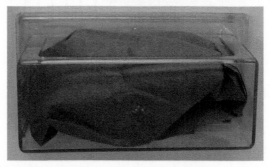

Fig. 8. Acrylic holder with brown bag of toys, food, or both.

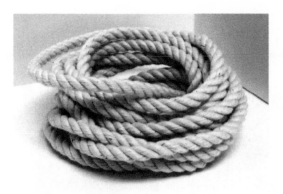

Fig. 9. Cotton rope can be used to create toys.

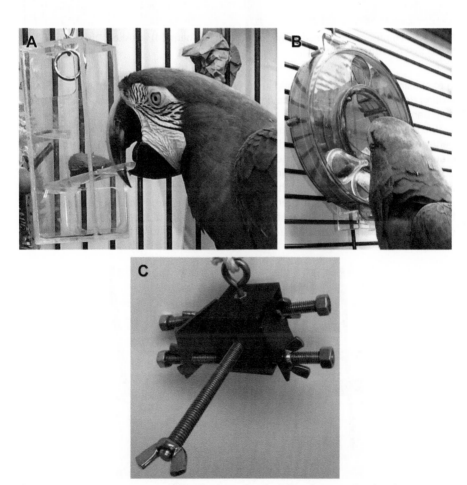

Fig. 10. Foraging toys range in difficulty from simple (*A*) to the complex (*B*, *C*).

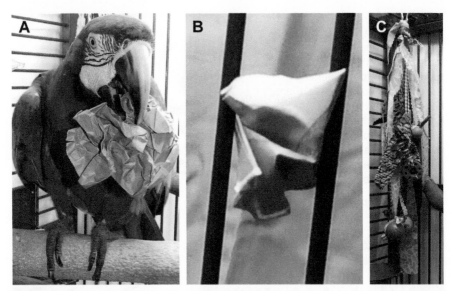

Fig. 11. Examples of homemade toys include brown bags (*A*), crushed Dixie cups (*B*), or beads tied on strips of cloth (*C*).

in exercising, foraging, or engaging in another enrichment activity. Enriching and promoting desired activities and behaviors help to either diminish or extinguish undesirable behaviors.

Two techniques for training include antecedent arrangement and target training with behavioral reinforcement. Antecedent arrangement is changing the environment to increase or decrease the likelihood of either desirable or undesirable behaviors occurring. Increasing or decreasing (or eliminating) stimuli that result in a behavior can be successfully used to teach and shape behaviors.

Target training is a means to train desired behaviors. Target training gives the trainer the capacity to tell the bird where to go (and what to do) to receive reinforcement. An effective reinforcement can be a treasured small piece of food that can be consumed

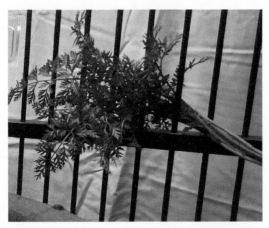

Fig. 12. Carrot tops or other greens can be woven between the cage bars.

quickly. The treat can be converted to a clicker in time. A target can be as simple as a wooden chopstick or as fancy as a commercially manufactured metal target stick. The bird is rewarded as it comes closer to the target, gradually requiring touching of the target to gain the reward. The target can then be used to guide and direct the bird to respond to the trainer's desired requests.

Punishment of an undesirable behavior, if manifested, should be structured through negative punishment, as opposed to positive punishment. Negative punishment is basically ignoring the undesired behavior; such a response does not reinforce inappropriate behavior and such behavior will ultimately be extinguished. Positive punishment is a response that causes pain or fear in the bird and is always an inappropriate response to any behavior. In addition, positive punishment can be a means of reinforcing those behaviors that are undesired.

SUMMARY

Pet psittacine birds are demanding companions. It is the avian veterinarian's responsibility to educate both pet owners and potential pet owners about proper care. The welfare and suitability of psittacine birds as pets are questionable. The welfare of the pet bird depends on the knowledge and motivation of the owner. Much is required to provide suitable mental and physical caretaking. Nutrition and housing are only the tip of the iceberg of appropriate care for pet birds. Providing for normal bird behavior, including foraging and socialization, is needed to meet their most basic needs.

REFERENCES

1. Engebretson M. The welfare and suitability of parrots as companion animals: a review. Anim Welf 2006;15:263–76.
2. Farm Animal Welfare Council (FAWC). RAWC updates the five freedoms. Vet Rec 1992;131:357.
3. Orosz SE. Clinical avian nutrition. Vet Clin North Am Exot Anim Pract 2014;17: 397–413.
4. Koutsos EA, Matson KD, Klasing KC. Nutrition of birds in the order psittaciformes: a review. J Avian Med Surg 2001;15:257–75.
5. Lisney TJ, Rubene D, Rózsa J, et al. Behavioural assessment of flicker fusion frequency in chicken Gallus gallus domesticus. Vision Res 2011;51:1324–32.
6. Morgan KN, Tromborg CT. Sources of stress in captivity. Appl Anim Behav Sci 2007;102:3–4, 262–302.
7. Newberry RC. Environmental enrichment: increasing the biological relevance of captive environments. Appl Anim Behav Sci 1995;44:229–43.
8. Clout MS. Foraging behaviour of glossy black cockatoos. Aust Wildl Res 1989;16: 467–73.
9. Echols S. Captive foraging DVD. Available at: AvianStudios.com. Accessed February 16, 2015.

Juvenile Psittacine Environmental Enrichment

Elisabeth Simone-Freilicher, DVM, DABVP (Avian Practice)[a],*,
Agnes E. Rupley, DVM, DABVP (Avian Practice)[b]

KEYWORDS

- Environmental enrichment • Juvenile • Nutritional enrichment
- Occupational enrichment • Physical environment • Psittacine • Sensory enrichment
- Social enrichment

KEY POINTS

- The juvenile time-frame is the first developmental stage during which most owners of psittacines have direct control over environmental enrichment.
- Social enrichment is facilitated by understanding the young parrot's communication signals, establishing and strengthening the human-parrot bond.
- Independent play is an important skill that must be learned by young psittacine birds, and toys from various categories should be provided for occupational enrichment.
- Nutritional enrichment includes variation in dietary offerings in type, presentation, and foraging opportunities.

INTRODUCTION

"Environmental enrichment" is a term that came into common use initially to describe modifications of the captive habitat of zoo animals. Because the concept is becoming increasingly applied to the living environment of companion animals, it is reasonable to wonder what environmental enrichment entails for psittacine birds. Because parrots are intelligent, highly social, emotionally complex animals, it is reasonable to ask "What is developmentally appropriate environmental enrichment for juvenile psittacine birds?"

Although environmental (particularly social) enrichment is of great import in the neonatal and preweaning psittacine, the juvenile time frame is the first developmental stage during which most owners have direct control over enrichment. A bird may be considered a juvenile once he or she is weaned, and before puberty (**Table 1**). The

Disclosure Statement: The authors has no affiliation with any products or service mentioned in this article.
[a] Avian and Exotic Animal Medicine Department, MSPCA-Angell Animal Medical Center, 350 South Huntington Avenue, Boston, MA 02130, USA; [b] All Pets Medical Center, 111 Rock Prairie Road, College Station, TX 77845, USA
* Corresponding author.
E-mail address: esimonefreilicher@mspca.org

Table 1
Ages of weaning, puberty, and sexual maturity for common species of companion psittacines

Species	Weaning (wk)	Onset of Puberty	Sexual Maturity (y)
Budgerigar	6–7	4–6 mo	1
Cockatiel	7–11	4–7 mo	1
Peach-faced lovebird	7–11	7–8 mo	1
Sun conure	8–9	9–18 mo	2
Green-cheeked conure	6–12	9–18 mo	2
Congo African gray	12–16	3–5 y	6
Eclectus parrot	14–16	3–5 y	6
Blue-fronted Amazon	12–16	3–5 y	6
Yellow-naped Amazon	15–18	4–6 y	7
Rose-breasted cockatoo	11–18	1–2 y	4
Umbrella cockatoo	12–18	3–4 y	8
Moluccan cockatoo	16–25	3–5 y	10
Yellow-collared macaw	10–12	1–2 y	4–5
Blue and gold macaw	14–22	4–6 y	8
Green-winged macaw	16–35	5–7 y	10–11

Data from Wilson L. 10 steps to a better relationship with your bird. Handbook of avian articles. EH Wilson; 2000. p. 14–7.

hallmark of this phase is increased athletic ability and a disinclination to cooperate, and may be the most common age of bird offered for resale by private owners.[1] From the onset of puberty until sexual maturity, a bird is considered an adolescent; physical, mental, and emotional needs for enrichment remain essentially the same during this time, although enrichment with potential for hormonal stimulation should begin to be phased out at this time.

In captive animals, the goals of environmental enrichment may be summarized as increasing behavioral diversity while (1) decreasing the frequency of abnormal behaviors, (2) increasing the range or frequency of normal (wild-type) behavior patterns, (3) increasing positive use of the environment, and (4) increasing the ability to cope with challenges in a more normal way (ie, resiliency).[2] For animals as intelligent as parrots, which are also possessed of such a rich emotional range, the list of goals for them may be expanded to include developing a sense of curiosity, a sense of well-being and happiness, healthy bonds to the family (human and nonhuman), and a certain degree of autonomy and self-care. In addition, owners should be aware that normal behaviors in a psychologically healthy psittacine bird are often loud, messy, destructive behaviors; a human who cannot tolerate living with a loud, messy, destructive creature should not try to live with a parrot.[3]

According to some behaviorists, environmental enrichment can be divided into five major types: (1) social, (2) occupational, (3) physical, (4) sensory, and (5) nutritional.[2]

SOCIAL ENRICHMENT

Social enrichment may be with either a conspecific or contraspecific (humans or nonhumans), and may include direct contact or noncontact, such as visual or auditory interactions.[2]

Social Enrichment for Healthy Interaction with Conspecifics

Parrot communication has been described as rich and subtle, and uses the whole body and nearly every feather.[4] Even if no conspecifics are present in the household, owners would do well to understand common communication signals (**Box 1**)[5] used by their young bird, because misunderstanding sexual behavior can lead to exacerbation of hormonal behavior, and failure to heed warnings of aggression can push a bird into escalation of the aggression, leading to a bite.[4] In contrast, accurate interpretation

---

Box 1
Common social behaviors seen between conspecific parrots

Aggressive warnings

Turn threat: turning to opponent with head and neck extended

Bill gape

Peck threat: pecking at opponent without contact

Wing flapping: facing conspecific with head extended

Sidle approach: rapid sideways approach

Slow advance

Rushing

Flight approach

Raised nape feathers with slightly lifted wings and growling

Beak clicking

Aggression

Peck: biting

Beak spar: beaks of both birds make contact

Wing smacking: swatting opponent with one or both wings

Submissive behaviors

Crouching

Fluffed feathers

Head wagging

Foot lifting

Avoidance

Affiliative behaviors

Allopreening

Allofeeding

Spending time in proximity

Reproductive behaviors

Blinking mimicry

Unilateral stretching of wing and ipsilateral leg

Adapted from Friedman SG, Edling TM, Cheney CD. Concepts in behavior: section I: the natural science of behavior. In: Harrison GJ, Lightfoot TL, editors. Clinical avian medicine. vol. 1. New York: Spix Publishing; 2006. p. 46–59; and Grindol D. Is your cockatiel being weird? In: Grindol G, editor. The complete book of cockatiels. New York: Macmillan Publishing; 1998. p. 99–104.

---

and appropriate responses to a young parrot's social signals helps establish and reinforce the human-parrot bond, and helps the owner guide and shape undesired behaviors. Although some behaviors, such as allopreening, are known to have frequency differences between the sexes in some sexually mature parrot species,[5] it is not known whether behavioral sex differences occur in juvenile psittacines.

Beak grinding or grating is another behavior that birds may exhibit when content,[5] and may or may not be affiliative. This soft continuous grinding noise should not be confused with the short sharp sound of beak clicking, which is a threat. An additional communicative sign is wing-flipping, which may indicate annoyance,[6] particularly in budgerigars and African gray parrots.

Careful observation of these communication behaviors facilitates introducing the juvenile parrot to other birds, and allows an owner to intervene before aggressive warning behaviors are replaced by actual violence. In single-bird households, veterinary clinic parrot behavior training classes can be one way to provide some degree of noncontact socialization among juvenile psittacines. The risk of transmission of infectious disease cannot be entirely eliminated in this type of setting, but the risk can be minimized by requiring each bird to have a minimum database including a physical examination, complete blood count, and *Chlamydophila* screening within the past year, and additional testing as appropriate for the individual's species.[7] A comprehensive guide for this type of class is available through the Association of Avian Veterinarians.[8]

Social Enrichment for Healthy Interaction with Owners

One author defines educating a bird as "showing that we love the bird, and are in control of the situation"[9] in a relationship of mutual trust and respect, much like that in which small children are ideally educated. The result is a bird that is confident, playful, and adaptable rather than fearful.[9] Interaction with humans is one of the "subjects" in which a young psittacine must be educated. Positive reinforcement training can be an excellent source of enrichment,[10] in addition to teaching the juvenile psittacine skills needed to live comfortably and happily with humans. A young bird should be taught to be comfortable with the owner approaching her cage, opening the door, reaching inside, and should be able to politely accept food offered by hand. If any of these common events are not yet comfortable for the young parrot, slow and gentle habituation is needed.

In addition, the young psittacine should be gently and gradually taught to respond to reasonable requests by the owner, including step up, step down, stay, and allowing touch to the wings, beak, and feet.[8] An additional behavior, allowing "hooding" in which the bird allows the owner's hand to be cupped over the head, is highly recommended to be taught because it can be used to shield the bird from perceived threats.[8] Much as for small children and dogs, compliance with certain requests should not be optional; the young bird should not be allowed to decide whether or not to return to his cage or step down from his owner's shoulder.[1] Following the establishment of these minimum behaviors, additional activities, such as trick training, can be continued throughout the parrot's life (**Fig. 1**). Consistent positive reinforcement for compliance with these requests facilitates learning.

Optional behaviors should be requested rather than commanded, to prevent confusion as to whether a behavior is expected. For instance, a young bird may be asked if it wants to come out of the cage; the interested bird will lean forward and possibly raise a foot, whereas the disinterested bird may move away or turn his back.[1] Like humans, psittacine birds experience the occasional "bad mood" and should not be forced to come out of their cages and interact at times when they are disinclined to do so.[11]

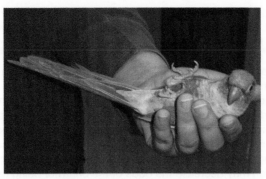

Fig. 1. This juvenile green-cheeked conure has already learned his first trick and is comfortable demonstrating it for strangers.

Many young birds can be accepting or even enjoy being touched and petted. One exception to this is during the juvenile molt, which is often heavy and uncomfortable. This may make the young bird unusually irritable.[1] Gentle stroking with a feather or a tooth brush may be more comfortable[1] and stroking in the direction the feathers grow is often preferred during molting to stroking against the grain, which may be enjoyed at other times. Owners of juvenile macaws and cockatoos are cautioned not to focus overly on petting and cuddling to the exclusion of other activities, because these young parrots sometimes grow to want and demand this attention to an extent that is beyond what most human time allowances can provide.[12] In addition, this exclusion of other activities by the juvenile, such as exercise and independent play,[13] can result in an adult parrot that is overly sedentary, emotionally needy, and unable to occupy himself.

Fearful or submissive behaviors should also be recognized by the owner. A fearful bird prefers to flee, biting only if she cannot flee[8] or when signals of distress are not responded to. Submissive behavior from the owner may help impart confidence in such a situation.[8] A timid bird may be raised higher to foster a sense of security[8] (it is usually perceived as safer to be above threats than at an equal height or below them). Our forward-facing eyes convey the stare of a predator; a fearful bird may find it more calming to be looked at with side-long glances as another bird might do, rather than a fixed or prolonged stare.

Contact calls are commonly used within flocks of psittacine birds to maintain communication while outside of visual range. This normal behavior is usually transferred toward the owner, and understanding it and responding appropriately can help decrease undesirable and excessive screaming. It should be understood that loud vocalizations, such as screaming, are also normal wild-type behavior for psittacine birds; owners should expect and accept a certain amount of this as part of their parrots' lifelong normal behavioral expression. The ring of a telephone or beep of an appliance may be interpreted and imitated by a young parrot as a type of "human contact call" because it is almost always answered.[3] Answering these and other pleasant sounds is imperative to teach the young parrot that a polite request is effective; otherwise owners risk teaching the young bird that only loud obnoxious noises are rewarded with a response.[3]

Some owners tend to think of contact calls as being an attempt to exert control over them by their parrot. Although this may be the case for some individuals, contact calls are a completely natural (wild-type) behavior for psittacine birds, and being out of both visual and auditory contact with a perceived member of her flock can cause great anxiety for a young parrot.[8,13] Proactive talking, whistling, singing, or humming by the owner to the bird, particularly when the human is out of sight, can help foster security and quell anxiety for the young psittacine.[7] In the household of one of the authors, the owners became so habituated to a particular whistled "flock call" that it became frequently used by the humans when visually separated from each other outside of the house, even though no pet psittacines were present.

Owners can facilitate quiet when it may be needed in the human environment by proactively providing enrichment that stimulates quiet activities, such as foraging or after-bath preening.[3] Active positive reinforcement of quiet enjoyment of play, foraging behavior, and preening is recommended to encourage the behavior to be repeated. Ignoring a desired behavior can be treated as a "punishment" by a highly social bird,[14] which may decrease the odds of the behavior being repeated.

Social Enrichment for Healthy Interaction with Nonpreferred or Nonowner Humans

Although it is common for companion parrots to prefer one owner over others in the household, this is not normal psittacine social activity[7] and should be discouraged. Preferred and nonpreferred owners can be identified sometimes even in the juvenile parrot, and this should be monitored and positive interactions with the nonpreferred owner reinforced. Sally Blanchard's "Warm Potato Game" in which the young psittacine bird is gently passed in a circle from person to person to interact positively with the bird is an excellent activity for teaching the parrot to understand that all "flock members" are valued and to be treated politely.[15] Opportunities for positive interactions with the nonpreferred owner can be readily created. The nonpreferred owner should be the one to take the bird to unfamiliar locations, both within and outside the home, including to the veterinary visit, because the strange and even sometimes frightening necessary experiences can make the nonpreferred owner seem all the more comforting and familiar.[7] When multiple owners are present at the veterinary visit, the clinician can make a point of finding out who the nonpreferred owner is, and allowing that owner to "rescue" the bird. Handling the bird in unfamiliar rooms in the home also facilitates the relationship. In addition, the nonpreferred owner can be the only provider of particularly favored treats, habituating the young parrot to look forward to that owner's presence. Any aggression toward the nonpreferred human should not be tolerated by the preferred owner, who should instantly respond with an angry look, say "No" in a quiet but displeased voice, and then turn his or her back on the bird.[16] If the nonpreferred owner is comfortable handling the bird, he or she should then quietly but firmly request several "step ups" from hand to hand ("laddering"); once the bird complies, positive verbal and visual reinforcement should be given, and no lingering grudge displayed for the biting.[16] Under no circumstances must the preferred person laugh when his bird bites another human. Although the sight of a small bird chasing a large human may understandably be seen as humorous, laughter is a strong positive reinforcement for psittacine birds.

Although most psittacines are understandably wary of unfamiliar humans, habituating the young psittacine to tolerate a stranger's approach to them or their preferred human is essential to securing the safety of the bird and the humans involved, because a frightened bird may flee and thrash and injure themselves, bite or otherwise attack the stranger, or even the owner in an attempt to drive the owner away from the stranger. Slow and gentle acclimation is the key to success in this endeavor, with plenty of positive reinforcement and careful monitoring of the young parrot's fear and stress levels to avoid generating heightened emotional tension, which works against habituation by the bird. Habituating the juvenile psittacine to tolerance of strangers can be vital to preserving long-term quality of life for both parrot and humans, because psittacine reactions to perceived interlopers are likely to be heightened and increasingly violent following puberty and during periods of hormonal activity. Desensitization should be initiated with frequent visitors first, followed by strangers; many birds may initiate contact themselves if first allowed to observe from a secure location.[11]

Social Enrichment for Healthy Interaction with Veterinary Professionals

Veterinary visits are another experience that most birds have occasionally throughout their lives. There are many components to this experience to which a young bird should be gradually and gently acclimated: the carrier, the car ride (or other mode of transportation), towels, and restraint.

Most young birds have not yet had an opportunity to become phobic of towels, although they may exhibit neophobia. Ideally, the towels used during the veterinary visit should not be highly patterned and should be of a neutral color, remembering that psittacine birds can see into the ultraviolet and infrared portions of the spectrum, so that a plain white towel might seem disturbingly bright to them. If the owner has acclimated the bird to towels at home, the bird may have a preferred towel that it is used to, and the owner should be encouraged to bring this to the visit.

Although the technique of quickly grabbing the bird with a towel from above and behind unfortunately may sometimes be needed in the case of an adult bird that is not tame (especially in many small species), this is not at all necessary and may be extremely frightening for the pediatric patient. Instead the towel may be offered to the young bird to explore and chew, and then gently wrapped around the bird starting from the front. Some avian behaviorists recommend speaking to the bird first, calmly explaining what will happen next.[17] Although different species and individuals may vary widely in how much of this monologue they may understand, it often does seem to have a remarkably calming effect. If the owner has already acclimated the young patient to towels, the owner may prefer to wrap the bird herself and hand him or her to the veterinarian.

Handling during the veterinary visit must be gentle and practiced; aggressive handling during the veterinary visit may precipitate phobic behaviors in psychologically sensitive species, such as rose-breasted, citron-crested, and triton cockatoos, African greys[17], and *Poicephalus* species. The practitioner and staff should enter the examination room calmly and quietly to avoid startling a bird, particularly if the bird is out of the carrier, because injury may occur.

Actual restraint should be as brief and gentle as possible. With many pediatric patients, this author often finds toweling and restraint is not always necessary. The pediatric patient may stand calmly cupped in an assistant's hand (**Fig. 2**), and allow a thorough physical examination including oral and caudal coelomic palpation, with the veterinarian softly speaking to the patient and maintaining eye contact. This author prefers to use words and sounds recognized and enjoyed by the parrot if these are known, or those commonly preferred by the species if the individual preferences are not known (eg, soft clicks for the African species). Additionally, sidelong glances with slow blinks are more psittacine and less threatening than the unblinking forward stare of a predator. Stethoscopes are occasionally somewhat alarming (possibly because of their resemblance to snakes or simply because they are novel), and if the bird is seen to withdraw or appear apprehensive, this author often stops and demonstrates the harmlessness of the instrument by tapping the bell lightly on her own cheek, and possibly that of the assistant, all while maintaining an encouraging eye contact and speaking softly to the patient. Once the young bird seems

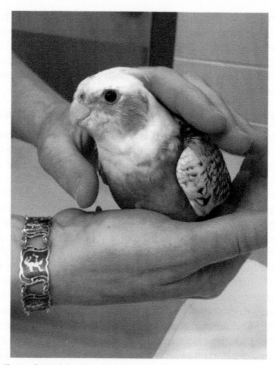

Fig. 2. This juvenile cockatiel is nervous for her first veterinary visit, but will permit full examination without requiring formal restraint.

to accept this, the bell of the stethoscope is lightly stroked over the bird's toes, until this too is accepted, and only then is auscultation of the heart, airsacs, and lungs attempted.

When returning the bird to the owner, allowing the bird to run across the table to the owner for comfort is helpful, and can strengthen the owner-parrot bond. However, for any juveniles that seem highly stressed by the examination, returning the bird directly to the owner sometimes seems to result in an association made by the bird between the owner and the visit, and phobic behavior toward the owner can ensue.[17]

OCCUPATIONAL ENRICHMENT

Categories of occupational enrichment include exercise-related enrichment and psychological enrichment, such as puzzles or ability to control or manipulate the environment.[2]

Exercise

Because psittacine birds evolved to fly a great deal every day, daily exercise is a necessity for the developing juvenile.[1] Exercise may include flapping and flying, chewing and shredding, and climbing and swinging. Like the young of any species, daily energy expenditure in appropriate ways can reduce the occurrence of "acting out" or expending energy in less desirable ways (screaming, pacing, or hyperactivity[1]). Habituating the juvenile parrot to these toys and activities early can be helpful later when puberty is reached, because hormonal fluctuations can increase the need to dissipate tension and energy.[18]

Objects to chew are important additions to any psittacine bird's home. If they are not provided, the bird will often try to find their own, which may be perches, cage covers, the owner's belongings, or her own feathers. One of the authors' Goffin's cockatoo, having destroyed her provided chew toys, which had not yet been promptly renewed, once released herself from her combination-locked cage, and made excellent use of a wooden entertainment center for this purpose. Both the chew toys and the combination lock were immediately replaced.

Less expensive materials can be readily provided to encourage chewing for development of masticatory muscles, fine and gross motor skills, and tactile exploration. Chewing is an excellent occupational "hobby" that most psittacines are predisposed to, and this should be encouraged. Many commercial toys exist for chewing, but can be expensive to continually replace once a young bird becomes proficient at chewing. A wide variety of chew toys should be provided, because individual preferences for specific substrates often develop. Nontoxic branches, old phone books, untreated wicker baskets, and tongue depressors are frequently used. Hobby stores can be sources of nontoxic wood in a variety of shapes and sizes, and cotton, sisal, and jute rope is readily found in hardware stores. Caution should be exercised in avoiding rope that is too soft, because these have been anecdotally associated with ingestion and gastric impaction, particularly in cockatoos. Many parrots enjoy chewing fabric, and this can be safely encouraged by choosing a tightly woven natural fabric, and carefully monitoring for and removing loose threads. Some owners invest a great deal in cage covers that cannot be easily destroyed, but no fabric cage cover is proof against a determined psittacine beak. (Cotton duck cloth usually takes little damage from small species, such as budgies and lovebirds.) This author prefers to use an inexpensive cotton bed sheet, and when it becomes too riddled with holes to serve its purpose it can be cut into short strips and tied into toys or cage bars for additional chewing opportunities. (The use of pinking shears to cut these strips is recommended to reduce loose fraying threads, which can be dangerous.) Vegetable-tanned leather is often enjoyed by many medium and large birds and can be found at leather hobby stores or on the Internet.

Novel items should be introduced periodically to the pediatric parrot. Neophobia, or fear of novelty, is a common stage most psittacine birds experience, although there may be a 2-month delay in age of onset for hand-raised birds compared with parent-raised individuals.[19] Food and items that will be part of the bird's every day existence should ideally be introduced before then to increase acceptance. This stage should be recognized when it occurs, because patience and more gradual habituation are needed to increase acceptance after neophobia has developed.

Wing-Clipping: Enrichment or Enrichment Reduction?

Flight in the wild serves a function, whether to procure resources, such as food, or a safe place to sleep or raise young, or to escape predators, none of which are required in a safe captive environment. In many parrot-human households, full or partial wing-clipping is required to ensure the safety of the parrot. In other homes, full flight is permitted to help provide escape from other pets that may be natural predators. Still other parrots are allowed full flight for behavioral enrichment, and some of these owners report that their birds seem subjectively happier and seem to scream less when allowed daily opportunities for flight. One author observes that wing-clipped birds seem less fearful and stressed by handling for the veterinary examination.[9] Regardless, wing clips should only be performed in the young psittacine after the bird has learned to fly and land with control. Although fledging in the wild generally occurs before weaning, the timing and duration of this period of learning plasticity varies somewhat among species. If this timing is not known, it can best be identified by assessing the young bird's skill and maneuverability in flight and landing. Allowing some time for flight in the fledging and early juvenile period provides physical and mental development that should be replaced with other exercise and spatial activities if flight is not provided.[12] Similarly, opportunities for vigorous athletic activity, such as climbing, flapping, and swinging, likewise should be provided, encouraged, and reinforced in the older wing-clipped juvenile psittacine.[12]

Many practitioners use the wing clip style often described as "modified sail"; however, the number of primaries and length of feather left should be modified based on species and body type. Short-tailed heavier-bodied birds, such as Amazons, caiques, Pionus parrots, and many African species, require a less severe clip than light-bodied long-tailed species, such as macaws, conures, cockatoos, cockatiels, and budgerigars. African species, especially African gray parrots, are particularly clumsy even as adults. Severe wing clips should be avoided in young birds of these species because this may exacerbate their natural clumsiness, and the consequent falls can increase fearfulness and associated behaviors. Additional clipping can be offered at no charge within 2 weeks of the initial clip, should the bird adapt and fly too well at home.[17] Alternately, a gradual wing-clip can be offered, particularly if this is the juvenile parrot's first clipping; four to six of the outermost primaries are clipped initially, followed by additional primaries on a subsequent visit or visits.[12] Advanced owners may also teach the young parrot who has already been conditioned to accept touch and handling of the wings to also allow clipping of a feather or two at a time without the need for restraint.

Following the wing clip (especially if it is the juvenile bird's first) padding the bottom of the cage with towels covered with newspaper is prudent to prevent injuries,[17] as well as keeping the parrot off of high places while adjusting to the wing clip. Ladders, rope walkways, and a variety of play equipment are recommended for exercise and to allow the young bird to avoid and seek out social interaction similar to the abilities of the flighted parrot.[12]

PHYSICAL ENRICHMENT

Physical enrichment may include the cage, cage furniture, toys, and accessories, and external home environment.

Cage

The cage should be appropriately sized for the species housed; ideally it should be wide and deep rather than tall. A good rule for cage size is for owners to purchase the largest cage they can afford and have room for. At least some of the cage bars should be horizontal rather than vertical, because climbing up and down vertical bars ("cage surfing") is a skill that takes some time to acquire and may be beyond the coordination of a young juvenile parrot.

Dishes

Although food and water dishes are not usually thought of as part of environmental enrichment, their color size, shape, and location can influence a young bird's attraction or aversion to food. One of the authors once treated a young cockatiel that was presented as an emergency for extreme debilitation because of starvation following replacement of his food cup with an otherwise identical cup of a different color. Novel foods or pelleted diets can be placed near favored perches to increase acceptance, whereas preferred foods may be placed in less desired locations, such as lower in the cage.

Perches

Perches ideally should be of varying materials, particularly materials that afford traction for very young birds because they are usually less coordinated than adults. Manzanita, which is very popular because it is difficult to destroy, is extremely slippery, especially when wet.[17] This may be exacerbated if the perch diameter is too large for the young bird to wrap its foot easily around. Additionally, prevention of destruction is not necessarily a desirable goal for perches, because chewing and shredding perches is a form of enrichment in itself. However, sand-blasted manzanita perches are available, which provide a better texture while remaining difficult to destroy.

Another factor that may contribute to perching insecurity is an overly aggressive nail trim, which reduces grip and may lead to falls and injuries and subsequent phobic behavior. Filing of the sharp tips of a young bird's claws may be preferable to clipping, to preserve claw length to facilitate a strong grip.[17] Because clipping and/or filing a parrot's claws will likely be performed many times over the life of the bird, it is important that early claw trimming experiences for the juvenile psittacine not be frightening, painful, or otherwise traumatic. In addition to gentle, respectful handling, the authors prefer to close the nail clippers slowly over the claw at the intended site to be trimmed, watching the parrot closely for facial expressions or bodily reactions that indicate discomfort. If these occur, the claw is not clipped at that location, but the clippers are moved more distally and the process repeated until the bird does not react. In this manner, not only is cutting the apt-to-bleed quick avoided, but the nails are also not cut close to the quick, which can be equally painful in some sensitive birds. Although some parrots are too stoic for this method to work, it is surprisingly effective with most juvenile and many adult birds. Similarly to wing-clipping, an experienced owner can also teach the young psittacine to gradually accept filing and even clipping of claws without the need for restraint. If a young bird has already had his claws overclipped or seems unusually prone to falling, a raised padded false bottom may be inserted on top of the cage grate to prevent injury[11] until the claws regrow or the young parrot becomes more athletic and coordinated.

Perches should also be of varying diameter; the dowels or plastic rods that come with most commercial cages can be thought of as "for demonstration purposes only," because the texture and unchanging diameter is hard on a bird's feet. A young parrot should become used to a wide variety of perches at an early age, which also provide exercise for feet and legs. Natural nontoxic branches can be acquired commercially or from nature. Fruit trees that have not been sprayed with pesticides are a safe choice, and can be scrubbed with a 10% bleach solution, thoroughly rinsed, and then baked in an oven for 10 minutes at 350°F to help destroy pests and pathogens. The owner is cautioned not to leave the oven unattended, because small thin branches in particular can ignite.

Materials other than wood can also make good perches and add to variety and enrichment. Twisted cotton rope perches are enjoyed by many species, as long as they are monitored for fraying and stray threads are frequently removed. In addition, a good quality cement perch can provide traction and desirable degree of roughness for feet, keep claws from overgrowing, and provide a substrate for beak cleaning and shaping by the young bird.

Toys

Independent play is an important skill that must be learned by a young psittacine. Toys may be grouped into four categories: (1) chewing, (2) climbing, (3) foot (or floor for smaller birds), and (4) puzzles.[1] Chewing toys are so designated to be shredded, destroyed, or manipulated with the beak. Climbing toys can include toys for climbing, swinging, or hanging on.[13] Puzzle toys require a bird to solve a puzzle or complete a task to receive a reward.[13] Although at least one toy from each category should be provided at all times for optimal enrichment,[1,13] crowding the cage with toys should be avoided because this limits space for exercise, and may be visually overwhelming to sensitive birds, particularly if brightly and variably colored. Toys should be periodically rotated into and out of the cage to provide variety and prevent boredom through overexposure to the same toys. Toy type, size, material, and suitability[13] must be carefully considered for the individual bird. Although a toy designed for a medium parrot may be thoroughly enjoyed by an intrepid lovebird, chewing substrates for a larger bird may be too hard for her smaller beak to destroy. Likewise, a toy designed for small birds may be given to a shy medium parrot; however, it must be able to safely withstand the more powerful beak of the medium bird unless it is designed to be thoroughly destroyed. Toys may also provide an outlet for aggression[1]; several species including Amazons, budgerigars, and cockatoos seem to occasionally interact very roughly with their toys, which may deflect aggression from other inhabitants of the home.

Not all juvenile parrots come into their human households already knowing how to play with toys. The owner may need to demonstrate this many times, by stopping when walking by the bird's cage and manipulating a toy briefly before moving on, or tearing up paper and happily throwing the pieces around with abandon.[20]

If the juvenile is fearful of new toys, they should be introduced gradually. A toy may be placed on a table a short distant from the cage, and casually played with and manipulated by the owner on occasion. When the bird exhibits curiosity, or at minimum a cessation of nervous behaviors, the toy may be placed closer to the cage. When the bird is comfortable with this, the toy may be hung on the outside of the cage, in a location that is below most of the perches, and away from food and water dishes so that any anxiety on the parrot's part does not make her reluctant to eat or drink. Once this is accepted, the toy may be placed inside the cage, preferably near a low perch away from food and water dishes. The entire process may take days or weeks depending on the degree of trepidation demonstrated by the bird.

Carrier and Cars

If a young psittacine's carrier and subsequent car rides are only experienced in conjunction with unfamiliar and often frightening experiences, such as grooming or veterinary visits, the bird will quickly develop an aversion to the carrier. Although grooming and veterinary visits need not be frightening, and every effort should be made to avoid it, in the beginning, the unfamiliarity alone may be frightening. For this reason, a young bird should be acclimated to the carrier as soon as they are comfortable with "step up" and "hooding," followed by being moved backward into the carrier, ending with "step down" and "stay."[8] Positive reinforcement can be provided by prior placement of preferred treats and a favored toy or two in the carrier. Initial placement in the stationary carrier may only last a few minutes for a nervous bird, and this can be gradually prolonged in subsequent sessions. Once the bird is comfortable being in the carrier for longer periods of time, moving the carrier can be introduced and made familiar, followed by short car trips. Visits to amenable friends' homes can provide a variety of novel enrichment experiences, including social, visual, and auditory.

Sleep Environment

Although the exact nighttime sleep requirements of psittacine birds have not yet been well-studied,[1] many authors recommend 12 hours of quiet and dark be provided for sleep.[1,21] Because this may be difficult to provide in the average home, acclimating a parrot to a "sleep cage" using any space that can be kept dark and quiet, including a walk-in closet or an unused bathroom, can be a prudent solution while a parrot is still young enough not to be habituated to sleeping in his daytime cage. This may become especially important once sexual maturity is reached, because a long diurnal cycle is commonly thought to be hormonally stimulating in many species of birds, and early habituation can help reduce additional stress and changes later during a very challenging time. Dim lighting may be preferred over darkness by some nervous birds at night, particularly cockatiels, which are subject to night thrashing.[5]

External Home Environment

Where the cage is placed in the home is often of great importance to the psychological comfort of the young psittacine. Although the confident highly social juvenile might prefer to be in the center of activity in the home, this may be overwhelming or intimidating for the nervous, sensitive young bird.[1] Such a bird may do better where he can see, hear, and interact with his humans, but not constantly, and where he can see them coming, away from a doorway where people may appear in a startling fashion.[1,7,13] Many such birds prefer a solid wall on at least one side of the cage, and possibly an area that is partially covered to permit hiding. This may be achieved with a cloth cover, branches fixed to the outside of the cage,[1] or even portions of old phone books threaded through the cage bars, or fabric strips tied in knots across the bars. Chewing on these elements provides exercise and occupational enrichment as well, and some birds thereby modify the coverings to achieve the level of concealment they find comfortable. Hiding places, such as wooden or cardboard boxes, can also be placed within the cage to provide additional security for the young parrot, and decrease repetitive stimulation of the "fight-or-flight" response.[11,17]

Windows can provide a form of entertainment and enrichment for parrots. Care must be taken that the view does not frequently show predators, such as hawks or neighborhood dogs. A young bird may feel more secure with only a portion of the side of the cage facing a window, while the other portion is against a wall to provide hiding space.[1]

Young parrots that spend all day in one place are more likely to be stressed by change or to become territorial.[13] Out of cage play-gyms, perches, or swings may be provided, preferably in a more active area of the home to provide exercise and social enrichment opportunities.

Another way the home environment can be used as enrichment is through an activity Kenneth Welle calls "House Tour."[7] Wild juveniles experience their environment while following parents and flock mates around, which exposes them to a variety of stimuli, food and other resources, threats, and so forth. This enrichment activity is designed to emulate this developmentally rich experience. Once the juvenile is acclimated to its owner and responds consistently to the "step up" command, he may be taken on the hand around the house, and various objects, sounds, people, and other pets can be introduced and named.

SENSORY ENRICHMENT

Sensory enrichment may be visual, auditory, tactile, olfactory, or taste oriented. A variety of sensory enrichment should be provided to juvenile parrots to facilitate brain development, prevent neophobia, and provide interest.

Visual Enrichment

Visual enrichment may be provided to parrots as soon as young birds open their eyes[12] and should continue to be offered to juvenile birds. Differences between avian and human vision should be taken into account when providing environmental enrichment. Psittacine birds can see into the fluorescent and ultraviolet spectra, factors that may affect food selection and mate choice.[22] This may impact a parrot's preferences and aversions regarding enrichment objects, which may seem to be of similar colors to human eyes. Many psittacine birds have distinct color preferences, and these may be discovered using a colored set of otherwise identical children's blocks or balls, or colored construction paper. Over several sessions, patterns emerge in which the bird frequently chooses or avoids specific colors.[1,23] Discovering a bird's color preferences and dislikes can be helpful in selecting toys, introducing foods, and even in housing and handling. For instance, one might choose not to place a cage near curtains, furniture, or a wall of a color to which the bird is known to be adverse, and wearing clothing, such as a hat or shirt in a disliked color, can provoke seeming phobic behavior toward an owner. Interactive games can be played with colored objects or construction paper where the colors are shown and named for the bird.[7] The game's interest can be further enhanced by using the model/rival technique first described for use in birds by Irene Pepperberg.[7,24]

Color can be added to enrich the bird's environment through external objects, such as pictures, home furnishings, and cage covers. As with any novel item, the young parrot's reaction to new additions should be carefully monitored, because aversive behaviors including screaming and feather destructive behavior have been anecdotally reported with the introduction of new paintings or décor in the caged bird's line of sight. Toys may be purchased in bright colors, or home-made toys can be colored with food or cake dyes, the latter of which can be painted onto objects for very bright hues. Many parrots seem to have a preference for pelleted foods of a certain color, and dying uncolored foods may increase acceptance, particularly if the food is novel.

A mirror is a form of visual enrichment commonly provided for smaller species, such as budgerigars, lovebirds, and cockatiels. The use of the mirror should be carefully monitored over time, and removed if courtship or aggressive behavior is displayed.

In addition to stationary objects, television and videotapes or digital recordings may be enjoyed by many psittacine birds, and may help alleviate boredom if the bird is home alone for prolonged periods of time. Nature shows (particularly those of wild parrots, and which do not feature predators) and gentle programming designed for small children are often particular favorites. Streaming computer videos are not recommended, however, because they refresh at a rate of approximately 50 to 95 Hz, well within the detection limit of avian vision.[22] For this reason, fluorescent lighting is not recommended for use in the pet parrot environment, because the noncontinuous light produces a stroboscopic effect[22] that may be startling or irritating. The author has occasionally observed young parrots (which have not been exposed previously to fluorescent lighting) during their first visit to the veterinary clinic freeze and crane their necks to stare at the ceiling lighting fixtures, with a facial aspect that closely resembles horrified fascination.

Auditory Enrichment

Auditory enrichment may include music, both instrumental and vocal, and nature sounds. Different species have different detection thresholds for frequencies that correspond to the frequency ranges of their contact calls.[22] Whether this corresponds to a parrot's preference auditory enrichment is unknown, but many owners report distinct preferences in music by their pet birds, as evidenced by vocalizing, bobbing in time to the music, and so forth. Such preferences can be highly individual, but in general budgerigars, cockatiels, and lovebirds often seem to enjoy higher-pitched faster music, African species enjoy "clicking" and popping sounds heard in some types of percussion, and Amazon parrots often seem to like opera. These preferences can be used in the veterinary visit as well, and clicks and sing-song speech do seem to entice and entertain receptive patients during their examinations.

In addition to enjoying a variety of sounds, a juvenile psittacine bird should be encouraged to develop pleasant vocalizations. Soft whistles, laughter, clicks, and words may all be taught at this time, whereas harsh, grating, or overly loud sounds are ignored. If a young parrot is of a species that is predisposed to acquire a human language, labels (names) for important family members and favored items are recommended to be taught. The owner should be sensitive to labels made up or chosen by the parrot, which may be an actual word (a friend's Meyer parrot refers to one of the authors as "Bird") or a contraction. For instance, Alex the African gray, known for his part in Irene Pepperberg's linguistic studies, used the term "banerry" for apple, a contraction of "banana" and "cherry."[25] The budgie of one of the authors would often make the request "C'mommy," a contraction of "c'mere" (come here) and "mommy."

In addition to teaching labels of known objects and people to a young bird, individuals that are phobic or species that tend toward phobic behavior (*Poicephalus* species, small cockatoos, Eclectus parrots, and African gray parrots[26]) can be taught an identifier, such as the word "creepy," to indicate objects that might be distressing or frightening. Other word choices exist, but are best if not used often in casual conversation and can be easily pronounced by the bird if she is so-inclined. In this way, the bird can be warned about upcoming events that might otherwise startle her. For example, an owner might tell the young bird, "I'm going to get out the vacuum now; it's creepy!" The aforementioned Meyer parrot was taught this word, and when a new bird named Cricket was introduced to the household, promptly pronounced, "Cricket's creepy!" The two birds never did become fast friends.

Tactile Enrichment

Psittacine birds possess numerous sensory receptors for touch in their beaks and skin, and variety and stimulation can be provided for enrichment and enjoyment of this sense. The bill tip organ in psittacine birds is exquisitely sensitive, and may lead to enjoyment of a wide variety of textures, shapes, and "crunch-factor" in toys, foods, and chewing substrates. This variety should be presented to the young psittacine as early as possible, so as to foster familiarity and decrease neophobia later in life.

Sensory receptors in the legs and feet are sensitive to temperature, pressure, and vibration.[22] A variety of perch textures should be introduced at a young age, and swings and bouncing perches, because these are excellent for exercise and for sensory enrichment.

Bathing skills must be learned by every young parrot, because they are vital to good feather and skin health, and can help with that oh-so-irritating heavy juvenile molt by softening the keratin sheaths of the incoming feathers.[1] Most human homes are much drier than a psittacine bird's natural habitat; even desert species are usually found within flying distance of water sources or other bathing opportunities.[1] Showering with the owner can provide an excellent social activity, and a good traction-providing commercial shower perch can greatly facilitate comfort and security for the parrot and human. If the young bird seems fearful, it may need to be introduced to this practice gradually, first by habituating to the room, which may be novel to the bird, then to the sound and sight of the running shower, then to being present during the owner's shower, and finally to the experience of getting wet. Bathrooms are usually full of hard surfaces on which a panicked parrot can easily injure herself, so great care must be taken not to push the young psittacine too quickly to avoid inducing injury or phobias.

Not every bird will safely acclimate to the shower, and some birds may have other bathing preferences, including the kitchen sink, a shallow dish in the cage, wet greens, or a spray bottle. Although some birds seem to enjoy being directly sprayed, many seem to find it noxious, and respond more positively to spray directed upward over them, to fall down gently on their bodies.

Following bathing, most birds engage in a prolonged session of self-grooming including shaking, scratching, stretching, and preening. This is sometimes referred to as a comfort behavior, because it seems comforting to the bird and because it occurs when the bird is comfortably at ease.[21]

Other Enrichment

Compared with humans with approximately 9000 taste buds, parrots have a poor sense of taste, with approximately 300 to 400 taste buds.[22] Most birds are thought to be able to taste salt and acid flavors, whereas the response to sweet seems to vary among species, with some parrots and budgerigars preferring sweet water to plain, and cockatiels preferring plain water to sweet.[22] Although most taste-related enrichment can also be considered nutritional enrichment, instant fruit-flavored drink powders have also been used by one of the authors to flavor chew toys and plain pellets for Goffin's cockatoos, and subjectively seemed to enhance enjoyment and even increase acceptance of pellets in a seed-only bird (at a time when fruit-flavored pellets were not readily available). Although it cannot be stated definitively that the flavor was the beneficial enrichment rather than the color the powder added, the drink powder did have the advantage of being able to be gradually reduced until no additional additive was needed for the pellets to be accepted.

Although birds have comparable olfactory abilities to mammals,[22] scent enrichment has not been well studied in psittacine birds. Because of their exquisitely sensitive respiratory systems, artificial scents or aromas that are not directly resulting from foods are not recommended because of the risk of respiratory irritation, injury, or toxic insult.

NUTRITIONAL ENRICHMENT

Nutritional enrichments may include variations in presentation, preparation, frequency and schedule of delivery, or in type including novelties, varieties, treats, and browse or foraging opportunities.[2]

Food Recognition

Offering a wide variety of foods to a very young juvenile is extremely important, even when the base diet is nutritionally complete. Wild parrots learn at a young age from their parents what foods are safe to eat, and from their own taste buds which foods taste good. By the time a fledged and weaned juvenile is acquired, that window of plasticity is already beginning to close. Continuing to offer a wide variety of foods during the early phases of a parrot's life maximizes the feeding options and possibilities for enrichment for the adult bird. One author recommends offering a pet psittacine new food items at least three times per week.[10]

Foraging

The value of foraging enrichment has long been recognized in zoologic collections, in aviculture, and increasingly in companion psittacine homes.[1] Because foraging is a natural behavior in psittacine birds, the young parrot should be encouraged to learn this skill to help develop mental abilities and provide constructive use of time. Foraging opportunities help a captive psittacine bird's daily time budget for feeding behaviors (30–72 minutes) more closely approximate those of wild birds (4–6 hours, or sometimes >50% of waking hours).[27] Foraging options may either involve hiding a food (opaque containers or toys); placing a food in a clear but difficult to access toy (puzzle toys); or interspersing food with inedible objects, such as large acrylic beads (impediments) or nut butter or nuts stuffed into the holes in cholla wood or holes drilled into nontoxic wooden branches or boards. Food may be provided in small amounts distributed among multiple feeding stations, or sequestered in toys that must be untied to access the treat, or must be raised from a cup suspended from a perch by a rope.[27] The "Captive Foraging" DVD by Scott Echols (Zoologic Education Network, 2006) is a valuable resource for ideas for owners.

Commercial foraging toys exist and can be supplemented by inexpensive homemade options, including empty tissue boxes, paper cups, and even crumpled pieces of paper. An additional benefit to foraging is that acclimating a bird to associate the foraging containers with food can help overcome nutritional neophobia. The cockatoos of one of the authors were highly averse to novel food items; however, once they came to greatly enjoy ripping open paper cups for food treats, they then began eagerly to devour the contents, even when the food presented was entirely novel.

AUTONOMY AND PUBERTY

Two stages that juvenile parrots go through can be particularly challenging and confusing for owners. These are the prepubertal stage of increased autonomy, and puberty. During the stage of increased autonomy (which may occur between 6 and 24 months of age,[20] depending on the individual and species), the young bird will naturally be growing toward a more adult independence. Activities that were once enjoyed, such as petting and cuddling, may not even be tolerated now, similar to a young boy rejecting these same activities that he may have sought after as a toddler.[3] If the juvenile psittacine has not yet been taught what behaviors are and are not acceptable, they are in increased danger of being rehomed at this time,[20] or in the case of smaller birds, consigned to their cages with little opportunities for interactions and experiences outside the cage.

During puberty, or sexual development, the young psittacines preferences and experience of events begins to develop into that of the sexual mature adult. Although young parrots may enjoy or at least tolerate being touched and petted, few psittacines seem to enjoy this into adulthood.[12] For those that do seem to enjoy it, close observation reveals that their enjoyment is increasingly sexual. A parrot is not a dog or a cat, species that have been bred and selected in many cases for the enjoyment of human petting and touch, and in the wild, long-bouts of allopreening rarely occur outside the mating season or pair bond. In addition, long petting sessions can themselves be hormonally stimulating. This can be extremely difficult for many owners to consciously understand well enough to alter their own behavior, either because they are treating the bird in the same manner as they are used to treating their mammalian companion animals, or because they have anthropomorphized and infantilized their pet bird. In the latter case, owners seem to find the following analogy helpful: "Your 3-year-old child may love to snuggle up with you, but if he does it to the same extent at the age of 17, the neighbors are going to start to talk." Nonhormonally stimulating interactions, such as spending time with and near (but not perched on) the owner, trick training, sharing meals as a family (ideally not warm mushy foods, which can mimic the sensory experience of courtship feeding), and showering together can all be substituted as social activities.

Sleeping huts and hide boxes should be gradually phased out during puberty, because the sexually stimulated young parrot will begin to see them as potential nesting sites, which can in turn be sexually stimulating. Likewise, any toy or perch that the bird regurgitates to or masturbates on should be removed. Dark periods of at least 12 hours overnight should be more carefully observed, and bathing can be increased because it can simulate a nonbreeding season, and provide distraction in the form of prolonged postbath preening.

REFERENCES

1. Wilson L, Linden PG, Lightfoot TL. Concepts in behavior: section II: early psittacine behavior and development. In: Luescher AU, editor. Manual of parrot behavior. Ames (IA): Blackwell Publishing; 2006. p. 60–72.
2. Young RJ. Environmental enrichment for captive animals. Ames (IA): Blackwell Science, Inc; 2003. p. 1–3.
3. Wilson L. When good parrots "go bad": tactics for integrating normal parrot behavior into the human household. Proceedings of the Annu Conf Assoc Avian Vet. August 5, 2007.
4. Friedman SG, Edling TM, Cheney CD. Concepts in behavior: section I: the natural science of behavior. In: Harrison GJ, Lightfoot TL, editors. Clinical avian medicine, vol. 1. Palm Beach (FL): Spix Publishing; 2006. p. 46–59.
5. Grindol D. Is your cockatiel being weird?. In: Grindol G, editor. The complete book of cockatiels. New York: Macmillan Publishing; 1998. p. 99–104.
6. Spadafori G, Speer BL. Birds for dummies. Foster City (CA): IDG Books; 1999.
7. Welle KR. Behavior classes in the veterinary hospital: preventing problems before they start. In: Luescher AU, editor. Manual of parrot behavior. Ames (IA): Blackwell Publishing; 2006. p. 165–74.
8. Welle K. Psittacine behavior handbook. Bedford (TX): Association of Avian Veterinarians Publication; 1999.
9. Hooimeijer J. Organizing a parrot walk/parrot picnic. Proceedings of the Annu Conf Assoc Avian Vet. August 26–28, 2003.
10. Shewokis R. Educating your clients on avian enrichment. Proceedings of the Annu Conf Assoc Avian Vet. August 10, 2008.
11. Davis C. Creating a happy and problem-free avian companion. Proceedings of the Annu Conf Assoc Avian Vet. August 30–September 1, 2000.
12. Linden PG, Luescher AU. Behavioral development of psittacine companions: neonates, neophytes, and fledglings. In: Luescher AU, editor. Manual of parrot behavior. Ames (IA): Blackwell Publishing; 2006. p. 93–111.
13. Welle KR, Wilson L. Clinical evaluation of psittacine behavioral disorders. In: Luescher AU, editor. Manual of parrot behavior. Ames (IA): Blackwell Publishing; 2006. p. 175–93.

14. Davis C. Behavior. In: Altman RB, Clubb SL, Dorrestein GM, et al, editors. Avian medicine and surgery. Philadelphia: WB Saunders; 1997. p. 96–100.

15. Wilson L. How to keep companion parrots from ending up in rescue. Proceedings of the Annu Conf Assoc Avian Vet. August 17–19, 2004.

16. Wilson L. The one person bird: prevention and rehabilitation. Proceedings of the Annu Conf Assoc Avian Vet. August 30–September 1, 2000.

17. Wilson L. Considerations on companion parrot behavior and avian veterinarians. J Avian Med Surg 2000;14(4):273–6.

18. Wilson L, Lightfoot TG. Concepts in behavior: section III: pubescent and adult psittacine behavior. In: Harrison GJ, Lightfoot TL, editors. Clinical avian medicine, vol. 1. Palm Beach (FL): Spix Publishing; 2006. p. 73–84.

19. Fox R. Hand-rearing: behavioral impacts and implications for captive parrot welfare. In: Luescher AU, editor. Manual of parrot behavior. Ames (IA): Blackwell Publishing; 2006. p. 83–92.

20. Wilson L. 10 steps to a better relationship with your bird. Handbook of avian articles. EH Wilson; 2000. p. 14–7.

21. Bergman L, Reinisch US. Comfort behavior and sleep. In: Luescher AU, editor. Manual of parrot behavior. Ames (IA): Blackwell Publishing; 2006. p. 59–62.

22. Graham J, Wright TF, Dooling RJ, et al. Sensory capacities of parrots. In: Luescher AU, editor. Manual of parrot behavior. Ames (IA): Blackwell Publishing; 2006. p. 33–41.

23. Harrison GJ. Perspective on parrot behavior. In: Ritchie BW, Harrison GJ, Harrison LR, editors. Avian medicine: principles and application. Delray Beach (FL): Wingers Publishing; 1994. p. 96–108.

24. Pepperberg IM. Grey parrot cognition and communication. In: Luescher AU, editor. Manual of parrot behavior. Ames (IA): Blackwell Publishing; 2006. p. 133–45.

25. Pepperberg IM. The Alex studies: cognitive and communicative abilities of grey parrots. Cambridge (MA): Harvard University Press; 1999. p. 33.

26. Wilson L, Luescher AU. Parrots and fear. In: Luescher AU, editor. Manual of parrot behavior. Ames (IA): Blackwell Publishing; 2006. p. 225–31.

27. Echols MS. The behavior of diet. Proceedings of the Annu Conf Assoc Avian Vet. August 17–19, 2004.

Ferret Wellness Management and Environmental Enrichment

Laurel M. Harris, DVM

KEYWORDS

- Ferret • Wellness • Disease prevention • Enrichment • Training

KEY POINTS

- Ferrets are a commonly kept companion mammal with specific husbandry and medical requirements for the maintenance of optimum health.
- Veterinarians have the opportunity to assist and advise ferret owners to best provide for their pet's needs.
- Psychological enrichment may be provided in many forms to maximize pet ferrets' overall health and well-being.

INTRODUCTION

Ferrets have been kept as companion animals for centuries. As intelligent, gregarious, socially engaging animals with a high metabolic rate and a propensity to develop serious, expensive disease processes, veterinarians owe it to them to assist owners in providing the best preventative care possible. The focus of this article is to provide veterinarians with the most up-to-date information to empower owners to provide an excellent quality of life for their ferrets in all stages of life.

LEGAL ASPECTS SPECIFIC TO FERRET OWNERSHIP

Ferrets are the most highly regulated of all common exotic small mammal pet species. Due to their potential as both a rabies vector and an invasive species in the United States, they are illegal in some states, counties, and municipalities. Clients should be advised to check their local laws and ordinances, preferably prior to acquisition![1] Owner heartbreak aside, confiscation and shelter placement can have dire consequences for ferrets. Veterinarians may be able to act on behalf of owners in acquiring

The author has no affiliation with any product or service mentioned in this article.
Wasatch Exotic Pet Care, Inc, 1892 East Fort Union Boulevard, Cottonwood Heights, UT 84121, USA
E-mail address: drlaurel@wasatchexotic.com

an exception under an exotic pet ordinance, but this should first include a frank discussion regarding the potential consequences if a petition is not successful. Furthermore, some state veterinary practice acts prohibit veterinarians from providing care for illegal pets and may require reporting of such by a veterinarian. Owners need to be advised that an illegal carnivore that bites a visitor to a home will face an unfortunate end should the bite be reported, regardless of vaccination status.

BASIC HUSBANDRY
Housing

Various housing options are possible for pet ferrets. If properly acclimated, they can thrive indoors, outdoors, or in a combination of both in most climates.[2] It is not advisable to allow ferrets to roam freely in the home. Their curiosity level, combined with a small, flexible, tubular-shaped body, enables them to both gain access to and escape from areas that pose little to no concern with many other pet species. They, therefore, should be housed in a secure, appropriate cage or enclosure and should only be allowed to roam outside the enclosure in a ferret-proofed area while under close supervision. Ferrets are especially fond of crawling into furniture and piles of laundry and seem to have a predilection for soft rubber items.[1,3] The author has treated many cases of "ferret versus recliner," clothes dryer–associated heatstroke, and television remote button ingestion. Ferrets are also not suitable for young children due to their ability to inflict a severe bite and the risk of blunt trauma from not-so-gentle handling.[3]

Examples of suitable indoor ferret housing are shown in **Figs. 1** and **2**. Multiple levels and vertical climbing options are suitable for younger ferrets. Older ferrets or those with medical conditions, rendering them less active or at risk of injury from routine play-related falls, should be allocated more horizontal space on a single level.

Commercial hutches or owner-constructed housing may be provided for keeping ferrets outdoors. As with any other species, enclosures must be escape-proof and adequately protect ferrets from predators and adverse weather conditions. Optimal environmental conditions include temperatures of 40°F to 77°F (4°C–25°C), humidity 40% to 60%, and 12 to 16 hours of daylight.[1,4]

Ferrets need a denning area and, in particular, appreciate hammock-style sleeping quarters. There are various commercial items to serve this purpose, although many owners choose to make their own. Ferrets tend to prefer warmth-retention fabrics, such as fleece. A simple, inexpensive hammock can be made with a hanging file frame (**Fig. 3**).

Most ferrets can be trained to use litter boxes. Litter boxes are most successful when placed in corners and cleaned frequently. For ferrets that would rather play in the litter or shove the litter box away from the corner, commercial potty pads placed in corners that ferrets have shown predilection for may be more successful. Owners should be advised that ferrets likely have a preference as to which corner(s) to use, and willingness to compromise on the part of owners results in less frustration for both parties.

Dietary

Dietary management is perhaps the most controversial issue in terms of overall wellness management of ferrets. Ferrets are obligate carnivores, with a very short digestive tract, lacking a cecum and ileocolic valve, resulting in a limited absorptive capacity and a need for a highly digestible diet consisting of high-quality animal protein and fat, with minimal carbohydrate and fiber.[5,6] Most sources advise 30% to 40% protein, 15% to 20% fat, and minimal fiber, offered free choice for most ferrets.[1,5]

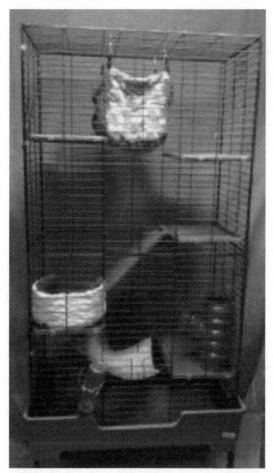

Fig. 1. Example of indoor housing appropriate for active, agile ferrets with climbing levels and multiple sleeping areas.

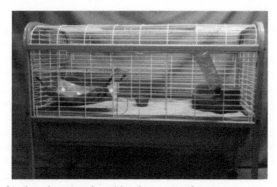

Fig. 2. Example of indoor housing for older, less active ferrets.

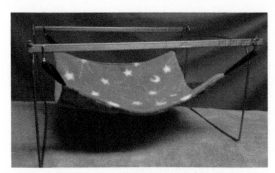

Fig. 3. Example of homemade hammock using hanging file frame.

Articles from 20 years ago listed appropriate ferret diets as cat or kitten chow as the base, with small amounts of vegetables and fruits.[7] Since then it has become accepted that there are critical differences in nutritional requirements between domestic felids and ferrets, hence the development of commercial ferret-specific formulated diets.[6] Many kibble-style diets have more carbohydrate and fiber than some ferrets can tolerate, which has led to the development of many forms and formulations. Additionally, some high-end feline diets seem to work well for some ferrets. In short, there is no one perfect formulated diet that can be recommended universally and owners need to be advised that they may have to do some experimenting to find which works best for their individual ferrets.[2,4] The author advises clients to find 2 to 4 brands with the appropriate composition of protein and fat and feed in combination. Because ferrets experience olfactory imprinting, it is wise to expose young ferrets to various foods early. Additionally, with the recent trend in frequent pet food recalls, this ensures that ferrets are not subjected to sudden diet changes if one of the main dietary components becomes unavailable.

Vegetables, fruits, and other high-fiber or high-carbohydrate foods, such as cereals, should not be fed as treats. High-quality ferret or feline meat-based treats are appropriate. Owners can be encouraged to use unseasoned home-baked meat treats. Whole-prey items can also be considered for supplementation because they mimic a natural diet in the wild, although many owners may find this an aversive option.

MEDICAL WELLNESS MANAGEMENT/DISEASE PREVENTION
Surgical Sterilization

A vast majority of ferrets in the United States are already surgically sterilized prior to availability to the public. Sterilization is mandated by most state laws, although it is legal for intact ferrets to be sold in a couple states and outside the United States. Owners who purchase intact female ferrets need to be made aware that they must be spayed or implanted to prevent estrogen-induced bone marrow suppression, which can be fatal. It is the rare owner who is be able to maintain an intact male ferret after the onset of puberty. For owners opposed to surgery, odor and aggression may be mitigated by placement of a gonadotropin-releasing hormone agonist implant, which has a reported effectiveness of 1 to 2 years. Because surgical sterilization has a causative link to adrenal gland disease (discussed later), it may at some point become the standard to leave ferrets intact and simply place implants as needed.[8,9]

Infectious Disease Prevention

Parasitism

Enteric parasites Screening for enteric parasites (in particular, coccidia) should be advised for all ferrets on initial examination, then once or twice yearly depending on risk factors.[7] Ferrets living strictly indoors may be exempted from routine fecal examination after initial assessment at a veterinarian's discretion, keeping in mind that potting soil can be a potential source of infection.

Ectoparasites Ectoparasite surveillance and prevention are the same as for domestic dogs and cats and vary regionally. Because ear mites are particularly common in ferrets and not always associated with clinical signs, it is advisable to screen for them on initial examination and after introduction of new animals.

Heartworm disease Ferrets are susceptible to heartworm disease. Minimal numbers of large adult heartworms affect a ferret's small heart earlier in the disease process in comparison to dogs and cats. Ferrets should, therefore, be maintained on heartworm preventative medication in heartworm endemic areas.[9] For strictly indoor ferrets in these areas, veterinarians should discuss risks with owners so that an informed decision can be made.

Viral diseases

Rabies As with other carnivorous mammals, ferrets are susceptible to and capable of transmitting rabies. Most government authorities that list ferrets as legal require rabies vaccination. There is one rabies vaccine that is licensed for use in ferrets.[10,11] Although this vaccine is labeled for use every 3 years in dogs and cats, it is to be given annually to ferrets.

Canine distemper virus Ferrets are highly susceptible to canine distemper virus (CDV). Because this disease is considered universally fatal in ferrets, vaccination for CDV should be considered every bit as important as rabies vaccination.[4] Choosing a vaccine in this case is not as easy. Various multivalent canine vaccine products were used successfully prior to the introduction of ferret-licensed monovalent vaccines. A safe and effective vaccine has been on the market for ferrets for years,[12] but availability from the manufacturer has become inconsistent recently and, at the time of this writing, the product has been on long-term back order. It is suspected that it may not be returning to the market and veterinarians again forced to choose from available canine products for off-label use. Although some practitioners choose not to vaccinate in the absence of a labeled product, the deadly nature of this disease necessitates that owners be involved in a discussion of all options available. If an owner elects to vaccinate with an off-label product, a vaccine with the fewest components should be chosen. Distemper/parvovirus combination vaccines are generally used by most clinicians. If owners choose to forego vaccination, they need to be advised to avoid any possible source of exposure—these include allowing ferrets outdoors with access to the ground; bringing any new dogs into the household; and walking in the house with shoes on after having visited a shelter, dog park, or other area frequented by a higher than average number of dogs of undetermined vaccination status. Vaccinated household dogs can bring the virus in on their feet as well. The myriad sources of exposure is generally sufficient to convince an owner that it is a wiser choice to vaccinate.

Vaccine reactions Ferrets are exceptionally prone to acute vaccine reactions. Because the risk of reaction increases with the number of vaccines given over time,[13] veterinarians may choose to offer antibody titer testing in place of simply continuing to vaccinate annually. Alternatively, most reactions can be prevented by pretreatment with diphenhydramine.[10] It is also a common practice to have owners wait in the office for 10 to 20 minutes after vaccination in the case of a reaction.

Influenza Documented since the 1930s, ferrets are exquisitely susceptible to many species of influenza virus, including human strains, so much so that they are used extensively in influenza research.[14] Mortality from the virus itself is rare and usually from secondary infections due to immunosuppression. Many clinicians routinely advise a course of broad-spectrum antibiotics as prevention when symptomatic ferrets present during flu season. Because annual vaccination is now highly advised for the global community, it is a wise practice to recommend vaccination for all household members in which ferrets reside. Veterinarians working with ferrets should also consider vaccination for themselves as well as recommending it for their staff members.

Ferret enteric coronavirus As the name describes, the ferret enteric coronavirus (FECV) causes mild to severe enteritis, commonly known in the lay community as green slime disease due to the passage of large quantities of bile pigment and mucus in the feces. Although the clinical signs can be severe, mortality from this virus is rare and generally a result of dehydration and secondary enteric bacterial infection if left untreated. The only true prevention for this disease is achieved by preventing exposure to an infected ferret.[3] Risk of FECV infection is a strong argument in favor of preintroduction quarantine with any new ferret. Although this is not a guarantee that resident ferrets will not contract the virus, an introduced ferret is more likely to shed the virus while subjected to the inherent stress of quarantine in a new home or shelter facility. Most clinicians advise a quarantine of 2 to 4 weeks.

Ferret systemic coronavirus Ferret systemic coronavirus was previously termed ferret feline infectious peritonitis due to its similar presentation to feline infectious peritonitis. It was initially speculated that this disease may have jumped species or that it was a mutation of the coronavirus causing FECV. Recent research has determined, however, that it is a distinct virus.[15] Therefore, it is unlikely that prior infection with FECV provides protection from this disease, which is eventually fatal. Owners should be made aware, however, that transmission is much more difficult, requiring intimate contact between ferrets (as with feline infectious peritonitis transmission in felids), and most exposed ferrets never develop the disease.

Helicobacter gastritis
Gastrointestinal ulceration is common in ferrets. Infection with *Helicobacter mustelae* is a common finding in many of these cases. There are several protocols in the literature for medical management and prevention of recurrence.[16]

Noninfectious Disease Prevention

Gastrointestinal foreign bodies
Ferrets are particularly prone to gastrointestinal foreign bodies due to their curious, investigative nature and small diameter intestine. As discussed previously, their predilection for soft rubber items poses a particular risk for obstruction. Dried fruit (banana chips, in the author's experience) has also been found to cause obstruction.[17] This finding can be used in the argument against feeding fruit as treats if an owner is not convinced by discussion of inappropriateness from a dietary perspective. Trichobezoars occur occasionally; therefore, over-the-counter hairball prevention medication

marketed for felines may be considered for use in ferrets with particularly fine silky coats or during times of heavy shedding.[3]

Gastrointestinal ulceration
With or without the presence of *Helicobacter*, stress has been documented as a significant cause of ulceration. Famotidine, ranitidine, or a similar H_2-receptor antagonist may be used to prevent excess acid secretion when a ferret is subjected to conditions that have the potential to cause significant stress, such as hospitalization, transfer to a new home, shelter placement, or loss of a companion.[4,10]

Insulinoma
Insulinoma is the most common form of neoplasia in domestic ferrets. Although inappropriate diet is not definitively linked to the development of insulinoma, the feeding of high-carbohydrate foods and treats can cause spikes in glucose and subsequent stimulation of insulin production. A high-protein, high-fat, low-carbohydrate diet may or may not help prevent insulinomas from occurring but certainly lessens the severity of signs associated with wide fluctuations in glucose and, therefore, insulin.[3] Additionally, one article discusses a possible association with the presence of mast cell tumors.[7] Whether real or coincidental, this potential association could be used as a reminder to clinicians to advise fasting glucose evaluation and may result in identifying cases of insulinoma prior to the development of serious symptoms.

Adrenal gland disease
Hyperadrenocorticism is a common disease in ferrets, so much so that clients who have done any of their own research are likely to have heard of the disease if they have not already had an affected ferret. Because surgical sterilization has been determined a causative factor in the development of this disease, this nearly universal practice in the United States has become controversial.[18] Because normal ultrasonographic parameters have been established in ferrets,[19] ultrasound can be used as a tool for screening, but prevention is preferable if young ferrets are seen by a clinician prior to the first luteinizing hormone surge at puberty. Prior to emergence of deslorelin implants, leuprolide acetate was under investigation for preventive use.[20,21] With the availability of deslorelin implants, potential prevention becomes a more convenient and economical option.[9] Investigation regarding the true efficacy of this practice is still in the early stages, but the general consensus is that it is currently appropriate to use these implants for preventive purposes. Owners may initially balk at the expense of placing an implant so closely after the series of first year vaccinations (which are often a surprise to new owners because many pet stores fail to disclose that young ferrets have only received the first in a series of at least 2, but more likely 3, CDV). For those owners receptive to this option, implants ideally should be placed in December or January of a male ferret's first year and in January or February of a female ferret's. Insufficient data exist at this time to suggest a definitive interval for replacement, although the labeled usage for therapeutic use is for 1 year. The author finds that a majority of owners who have had experience with adrenal gland disease and its various sequelae are rarely hesitant to invest in potential prevention.

Lymphoma
Lymphoma is common in ferrets, with no true preventative aside from good nutrition and a healthy environment. This is a primary reason for regular veterinary examinations, with the goal of identifying this universally devastating disease in the early stages and initiating treatment prior to the onset of severe clinical signs.

Urolithiasis

Urolithiasis occurs occasionally in ferrets as with dogs and cats. For struvite uroliths, dietary manipulation is controversial. Diets intended to decrease stone formation in dogs and cats are lower in protein than what is appropriate for ferrets.[7] Cystine urolithiasis seems to be emerging as the most common form of urolithiasis in ferrets in the United States. Because it has been determined to have a familial pattern of inheritance in both humans and dogs, this may be the case in ferrets as well. Cystine urolithiasis is much more common in the United States, where extensive inbreeding is a problem. This is compelling evidence that there may be a hereditary factor.[22] It is too soon, however, to rule out diet as a factor and a combination of the 2 may prove causative. At this time, the only preventive option for urolithiasis in ferrets is to maintain adequate hydration and avoid feeding any diets that have been associated with cases of cystine urolithiasis.[23]

Geriatrics

With their short life span and rapid metabolism, ferrets are considered by most veterinarians to be middle-aged at approximately 3 years of age. If an owner has not already been convinced that twice-yearly examinations are appropriate, this is good a time to approach this discussion, giving clinicians the potential to identify diseases prior to the point at which owners are likely to notice a problem. Blood work should be advised at this time, at least annually. Dental and periodontal disease generally begins to develop at this age, so regular dental prophylaxis should be performed or at least discussed with owners.[10] If changes in the teeth referable to diet (abrasion from hard kibble or calculus deposition secondary to soft or high-carbohydrate diets) are observed, dietary management/changes can be discussed with owners in addition to any recommendations for transitioning to a diet more appropriate for a senior ferret.[24]

Regarding dramatic weight and coat loss, it is normal for ferrets to experience weight loss of up to 40% during spring or summer (timing may vary by geographic locale). The winter coat also normally sheds at this time. These changes should not be confused with hyperadrenocorticism or other diseases for which these findings can be characteristic. If ferrets are active and eating well and there are no additional findings on physical examination, owners should be advised to monitor ferrets and expect weight gain and hair regrowth. If owners are not comfortable monitoring on their own, they can be given the option to stop in an office weekly for weight checks, during which time a staff member can also briefly evaluate the ferret.

PSYCHOLOGICAL HEALTH MANAGEMENT

Wellness management for a companion animal is not complete without thorough consideration for that animal's psychological needs. The younger generation of exotic companion animal veterinarians may not have experienced the zoos of old, with sterile cubical-type enclosures, their inhabitants ceaselessly pacing or developing other bizarre stereotypic behaviors. Environmental enrichment in zoos has developed over the past 3 to 4 decades to include not only more spacious and naturalistic enclosures but also opportunities for captive animals to engage in activities consistent with their natural history in the wild. Similar environmental manipulation can provide pet ferrets with mental stimulation and outlets for their need for activity. Owners who are committed to taking the time to implement as least some of the recommended measures ultimately have a more enjoyable experience with their companion ferrets.

Environmental Enrichment

Provision of environmental enrichment is unlimited in terms of options. Owners should be encouraged to use their imagination in developing ideas to keep their ferrets busy and engaged and to disperse their natural energy in a healthy and appropriate manner. The common hazards, most of which are discussed previously, need to be considered: temperature extremes, escape, falls, and exposure to harmful substances or items should be brought to owners' attention when initiating this discussion. Common sense must never be assumed by veterinarians when advising clients.

Wild polecats, as most other mammalian species, are solitary by nature, with adults encountering one another only for breeding or territory maintenance purposes. Thus it is appropriate for pet ferrets to be kept singly.[2,25] That said, a greater responsibility resides with owners as the sole providers of all options for healthy activity. Domestic ferrets, when given the opportunity, usually accept and engage with other ferrets. A huge proportion of their energy can be exhausted in this sort of social setting with no more investment from owners other than to be present to supervise, then sit back and enjoy the show. Well-socialized ferrets stalk, pounce, chase, and wrestle, engaging in an exhibition of their natural predatory, territorial, and breeding behaviors. Bonded ferrets usually prefer to sleep piled on top of one another. When choosing to house multiple ferrets together, most rescue organizations advise keeping a minimum of 3 ferrets, because they have a tendency to develop extremely strong bonds and the loss of a single companion can have detrimental consequences for a surviving ferret. Many ferrets experience grieving as is seen in species that mate for life, the severity of which can require hospitalization for prolonged anorexia, relapse of a previously controlled *Helicobacter* gastritis, or stress-induced gastrointestinal ulceration. Methods of introduction are beyond the scope of this article and are discussed in detail elsewhere.[25,26]

A ferret's housing in and of itself can be a source of enrichment. The primary living quarters can be as elaborate as desired to keep the ferret busy, or playpen-type areas can be constructed separately from the primary cage.[2] Ease of access to properly clean enclosures and devices should be considered.

A list of toys, devices, and play scenarios is provided in **Box 1** but is by no means an exhaustive list of options available to provide both mental stimulation and an outlet for physical energy for ferrets.

Training

Operant conditioning, also known as positive reinforcement training, is another form of enrichment that is widely used in zoologic institutions and can be integrated into a companion animal's enrichment repertoire. Environmental enrichment and training have been determined so beneficial for zoo and laboratory animals that they have been federally mandated in the United States for many mammalian species, requiring formal documentation of training plans and recordkeeping of daily training sessions for primates, in particular.[27]

Any client who expresses interest in any form of environmental enrichment can be introduced to the idea of training, although not every client has the capability of taking a ferret's enrichment to this next level. Because it has been determined that ferrets operate on the same cognitive level as domestic canines, any training resources intended for use with dogs may be applied to working with ferrets.[28] For those who are interested in pursuing training with a ferret, there are many resources available, from traditional book form, which includes the basic psychological principles behind training procedures,[29] to Internet videos produced by both amateur and professional

Box 1
Ferret enrichment devices and ideas

- Dig boxes/ball pits
  - Fill cardboard or deep plastic sweater box with packing peanuts, shredded paper, small plastic balls, uncooked rice, play sand, potting soil, etc.
- Commercially marketed toys for ferrets
- Manipulative toys
  - Commercial cat toys—crinkle balls, bell balls, mouse toys, feather teasers
  - Remote-control toys, small toy cars for chase-and-pounce play
  - Suspend a toy/ball from ceiling to just within ferret's reach with string or elastic for bungee activity.
  - Glue various objects inside plastic Easter eggs: bells, rice, dry beans, pea gravel, single large stone or marble.
  - Seal small cardboard boxes or paper grocery bags with various objects inside, with holes cut for ferret to explore.
- Water activity
  - Place 2–3 cm of water in a bathtub or kiddie pool, add various floating toys. Provide access for ferret to climb in and out at will.
  - Some ferrets enjoy swimming in deeper water—supervise at all times in this case.
- Tunnel and maze activity
  - Create tunnels with polyvinyl chloride pipe, dryer hose, industrial tubing, or cylindrical boxes.
  - Create mazes with large/appliance boxes, incorporating tunnels, or running tunnels around and under furniture. Multilevel tunnels can be made with flexible tubing, such as dryer hose.
- Owner-engaged activities
  - Gentle tug-of-war
  - Hide-and-seek, stalk and chase around furniture and tunnels
  - "Magic carpet ride" on a towel
- Olfactory enrichment
  - Purchase various wildlife species (deer, fox, etc.) scents from hunting supply retailers; rub small amount on toys or objects in favorite play areas.
  - Rub dried herbs or spices on items.[a]
- Food-related enrichment—note: food enrichment need not be restricted to treats! It is completely acceptable to use a ferret's entire daily diet presented in enrichment devices. This method may reduce the risk of obesity associated with overfeeding of treat items.
  - Rub FerreTone on nonporous toys and items.
  - Place a few pieces of food in a cardboard food carton; cut small holes to make ferret dig and shred the carton.
  - Place pieces of food in a plastic water or soft drink bottle with a small opening, leaving cap off. Let ferret roll the bottle around until the treat falls out.

[a] Some owners wish to use essential oils; in this case, owners should be advised that only miniscule amounts be used, not in combination, and that ferrets should be monitored for any adverse effects during first use.
Adapted from Fisher P. Ferret behavior, exotic pet behavior. Exotic DVM Magazine 2006;6(6):20.

trainers.[30,31] In this day and age where anyone can post anything to the Internet, veterinarians should personally review any training resources advised to ensure that proper and humane practices are promoted.

Because many clients are better convinced when they can see something tangible in a veterinary office, veterinarians may want to become personally practiced in 1 or 2 simple training scenarios. Getting ferrets to voluntarily step onto a scale or station for a vaccination without being forcibly restrained can be strong reinforcer for owners, most of whom appreciate a more positive experience in the veterinary office.

For veterinarians who are motivated to incorporate training into daily patient management, this can have a dramatically positive effect on patients in terms of decreased stress and conditioned fearful responses. Owners in turn may be more responsive to advice regarding more frequent veterinary wellness visits, screening diagnostics, and so forth, and the stress level on the veterinary staff is reduced in knowing that patients are participating in their care as opposed to submitting to it.

Veterinary support staff can be particularly valuable in becoming involved with training-based enrichment programs. Veterinary technicians or assistants who have an interest in behavior and training or simply wish to be more involved in providing humane patient care can be delegated the responsibility of setting up and maintaining a training program, teaching the basics to clients, and providing ongoing coaching and support.[32] As with training intended for owner use with ferrets at home, resources are readily available for training for patient participation in various veterinary procedures.[33]

A significant proportion of ferrets with white coat coloration, especially involving facial markings, may have congenital deafness.[34] These ferrets should be identified prior to initiation of training so that appropriate cues and bridges, such as hand signals, can be tailored to a ferret unable to hear a clicker, whistle, or a voice.

SUMMARY

Veterinarians seeing companion ferrets in practice have the opportunity to maximize their patients' quality of life by taking a proactive approach to the prevention of commonly encountered illnesses and hazards. Quality ferret care can be further elevated by the provision of environmental enrichment, for which countless options are possible. An open, honest relationship with receptive owners can result in dramatic elevation of the pet–owner bond.

REFERENCES

1. Kiefer K, Johnson D. What veterinarians need to know about ferrets. Exotic DVM Magazine 2006;8(2):38–43.
2. Lewington J. Ferret husbandry, medicine and surgery. Edinburgh (United Kingdom): Reed Educational and Professional Publishing; 2000. p. 26–74.
3. Powers L, Brown S. Ferrets, ferrets, rabbits and rodents clinical medicine and surgery. 2012. p. 1–26.
4. Fox J. Biology and diseases of the ferret. Philadelphia: Lea & Febiger; 1988. p. 140–257.
5. Bell J. Ferret nutrition. Vet Clin North Am Exot Anim Pract 1999;2(1):169–92.
6. Willard T. Exotic animal nutrition-ferrets. Exotic DVM Magazine 2002;4(4):36–7.
7. Rosenthal K. Ferrets. Vet Clin North Am 1994;24(1):2–15.
8. van Zeeland Y, Pabon M, Roest J, et al. Use of a GnRH agonist implant as alternative for surgical neutering in pet ferrets. Vet Rec 2014;175(3):66.
9. Suprelorin F (deslorelin acetate 4.7 mg implant) Virbac AH, Inc, Ft. Worth, TX 76137, 855–647-3747.

10. Hoppes S. The senior ferret. Vet Clin North Am Exot Anim Pract 2010;13(1): 107–10.
11. Imrab 3/Imrab3 TF, Merial, Inc, Athens, GA 30601.
12. Purevax CDV, Merial, Inc, Athens, GA 30601.
13. Moore G, Glickman N, Ward M, et al. Incidence of and risk factors for adverse events associated with distemper and rabies vaccine administration in ferrets. J Am Vet Med Assoc 2005;226(6):909–12.
14. Pignon C, Mayer J. Zoonoses of ferrets, hedgehogs, and sugar gliders. Vet Clin North Am Exot Anim Pract 2011;14(3):541–2.
15. Yutaka T, Shohei M, Maeda K. Genetic characterization of coronaviruses from domestic ferrets, Japan. Emerg Infect Dis 2014;20(2):284–7.
16. Carpenter J. Exotic animal formulary. 4th edition. St. Louis (MO): Elsevier; 2013. p. 561–80.
17. Johnson D. Online forum: ferret GI obstruction with dried fruit. Exotic DVM Magazine 2007;9(2):18.
18. Shoemaker NJ, Schuurmans M, Moorman H, et al. Correlation between age at neutering and age of onset of hyperadrenocorticism in ferrets. J Am Vet Med Assoc. 2000 Jan 15;216(2):195–7.
19. Kuijten A, Schoemaker N, Voorhout G. Ultrasonographic visualization of the adrenal glands of healthy ferrets and ferrets with hyperadrenocorticism. J Am Anim Hosp Assoc 2007;43(2):78–84.
20. Johnson-Delaney C. Ferrets as I see them. Exotic DVM Magazine 2009;11(1): 11–2.
21. Lupron, TAP pharmaceuticals.
22. Nwaokoric E, Osborn C, Lulich J, et al. Epidemiological evaluation of cysteine urolithiasis in domestic ferrets (Mustela putorius furo): 70 cases (1992–2009). J Am Vet Med Assoc 2013;242(8):1099–103.
23. Fisher P. Cystine urolithiasis in the ferret (Mustela putorius furo). Proc. Assoc Exotic Mammals. 2014.
24. Hoefer H, Fox J, Bell J. Gastrointestinal diseases. In: Ferrets, rabbits and rodents clinical medicine and surgery. St. Louis (MO): Elsevier; 2012. p. 27–31.
25. Fisher P. Ferret behavior. In: Exotic pet behavior. St. Louis (MO): Saunders/Elsevier; 2006. p. 163–205.
26. Staton V, Crowell-Davis S. Factors associated with aggression between pairs of domestic ferrets. J Am Vet Med Assoc 2003;222(12):1709–12.
27. Brown S. Small mammal training in the veterinary practice. Vet Clin North Am 2012;15(3):469–85.
28. Hernadi A, Kis A, Turcsan B, et al. Man's underground best friend: domestic ferrets, unlike the wild forms, show evidence of dog-like social-cognitive skills. PLoS One 2012;7(8):e43267.
29. Pryor K. Don't shoot the dog!: the new art of teaching and training. Lydney (United Kingdom): Ringpress Books Ltd; 2002.
30. Joey the Trained Ferret, Youtube video collection (74 videos), Jul 28, 2013.
31. SuperSonic Ferrets, Youtube video collection (115 videos), Dec 30, 2013.
32. Schaeffer A. Technicians and exotic animal training. Vet Clin North Am Exot Anim Pract 2012;15(3):523–30.
33. Mattison S. Training birds and small mammals for medical behaviors. Vet Clin North Am Exot Anim Pract 2012;15(3):488–99.
34. Piazza S, Abitbol M, Gnirs K, et al. Prevalence of deafness and association with coat variations in client-owned ferrets. J Am Vet Med Assoc 2014;244(9): 1047–52.

Small Exotic Companion Mammal Wellness Management and Environmental Enrichment

Ⓐ CrossMark

Anthony A. Pilny, DVM, DABVP (Avian)

KEYWORDS

- Wellness • Preventative medicine • Environmental enrichment • Education
- Exotic mammal

KEY POINTS

- Preventative veterinary medical care is an important part of keeping exotic companion mammals healthy.
- Veterinarians should encourage annual or biannual wellness visits for all pets.
- Environmental enrichment is necessary for a pet's psychological health and well-being.
- Clients must be educated on proper husbandry, diet, and enrichment for mental stimulation to decrease the likelihood of medical problems of small exotic mammals.

INTRODUCTION

Preventative veterinary medicine is defined as the science aimed at preventing disease in captive animals. It can also be simply defined as doing all one can to decrease the likelihood of developing medical conditions that could have been otherwise avoided. All too often the concepts of environmental enrichment, socialization, and exercise for small exotic pet mammals are ignored as many of these pets, such as guinea pigs, ferrets, hamsters, chinchillas, and rats, will live most of their lives in cages or tanks with little regard given to their mental and physical stimulation. Without education on wellness care, inappropriate diets and poor husbandry practices lead to animals becoming obese, lazy, and less likely to interact and provide pleasure as pets. Constant confinement without enrichment will lead to stress as well as certain otherwise avoidable behavioral and health problems. Veterinarians treating small exotic mammals should not only be familiar with the species' native habitats, lifestyles, and social interactions but also how to educate clients to ensure these unique pets

The author has no affiliation with any product or service mentioned in this article.
The Center for Avian and Exotic Medicine, 562 Columbus Avenue, New York, NY 10025, USA
E-mail address: apilny@avianandexoticvets.com

receive proper care during veterinary visits. It is a misconception that these animals are maintenance free because they do not need to be walked or mentally and physically enriched. Exotic pets living in our homes are usually captive bred and depend entirely on their human caretakers for food and exercise and often in need of social time and companionship.

VETERINARY WELLNESS VISITS

Any veterinarians treating small exotic mammals must encourage clients to schedule regular wellness visits. Many pet owners still think they should or choose to only seek veterinary care when the pet is sick or in need of medical intervention, which is a huge oversight. The new pet or postadoption/postpurchase visit is one of the most important as an opportunity to educate clients on everything they should be aware of to keep their pet healthy. Suggestions of diet, training, and general care as well as reliable Web sites and hospital-prepared care sheets and handouts can be provided. The wellness visit is a chance to discuss new diets or current research, monitor the pet's weight, and perform routine blood tests, fecal testing when appropriate, and radiographs for earlier diagnosis and prevention of disease. It also allows the veterinary to guide pet owners to trusted Web sites and correct any misconceptions they may have read or heard about their pet. Discussion of spaying and neutering is also imperative during these visits and should not be overlooked. Mammary masses in rats, ovarian cystic disease in guinea pigs, and uterine adenocarcinomas in rabbits are just a few examples of preventable conditions that can be avoided with elective ovariohysterectomy. All too often veterinarians are faced with the death of or having to perform euthanasia of a pet with an otherwise preventable disease, meaning one that might have been avoided if the client had elected more responsible veterinary care. Lastly, these visits are essential in establishing a relationship that allows the clients to call or e-mail with questions or concerns and use the veterinary hospital for services, such as nondoctor grooming and boarding where offered. Unfortunately, convincing pet stores and breeders to recommend postpurchase or postadoption veterinary visits remains a challenge.

SPECIES-SPECIFIC VETERINARY RECOMMENDATIONS

- Rabbits, especially from pet stores or breeders, should have a fecal ova/parasite check for coccidia and treated accordingly. There are no currently approved vaccinations for rabbits in the United States at this time.
- Guinea pigs and rats should be evaluated for pediculosis as lice are commonly seen. Checking for the presence of nits (louse eggs) is also necessary and treated accordingly.
- Ferrets need vaccinations for rabies and distemper virus according to both local and state law and veterinarian recommendations for need. Currently, there is no approved distemper vaccination available for ferrets.
- Chinchillas should be tested for giardia infection and treated accordingly. Also, fur loss or signs of possible dermatophytosis should be assessed.
- All small mammals, but rabbits and chinchillas particularly, should have a full oral examination to evaluate for dental disease, such as malocclusion or other congenital anomalies.
- Elective castration of male rabbits will markedly decrease the likelihood of urine scent marking and humping behaviors in males and dominance behaviors of female rabbits. Spaying and neutering are important for some pets' ability to cohabitate.

- There should be an in-depth review of dietary practices and recommendations, especially for sugar gliders.
- Body weight and growth rates should be evaluated in all small exotic mammals.

ENVIRONMENTAL ENRICHMENT

By definition, environmental enrichment, also termed *behavioral enrichment*, is the husbandry principle that should enhance the quality of pet care by providing the environmental stimuli necessary for optimal psychological well-being (**Table 1**). The goals are to improve an animal's physical and psychological health by increasing the species-specific normal behaviors, providing better utilization of the environment, and, thus, preventing or reducing the frequency of aberrant behaviors. Environmental enrichment should not be seen as an option in pet exotic mammal care because providing appropriate items to enhance the animal's captive environment is necessary to meet their emotional needs. Because most zoos, marine mammal parks, and sanctuaries have had to evolve their captive husbandry protocols to better meet these vital needs, individual pet owners must do the same. The following are the main groups of enrichment:

- *Occupational/environmental*: enhancing the pet's habitat in ways that change or add complexity
- *Social*: providing the ability to live with and interact with other animals
- *Dietary/nutritional*: encouraging animals to investigate and work for their food by using different methods of food presentation
- *Sensory*: stimulating animals' senses (visual, olfactory, taste)
- *Manipulation*: promoting investigatory play by providing items that can be manipulated by the paws, feet, tail, mouth, and so forth; requiring a pet to solve problems to access food or other rewards with puzzles/games
- *Training*: training animals with positive reinforcement or similar methods

GENERAL CONCEPTS
The Cage

Because many small exotic pet mammals live in cages or tanks, each should have the largest cage that owners can afford, maintain, and have room for. Because many exotic mammals spend most of their lives in cages, extra inches or feet make a big

Table 1
Enrichment based on natural history and typical behaviors

Natural History	Behavior	Equipment	Enrichment
Food quest	Foraging, digging, eating	Box of paper litter or tub of soil	Work to find treats, dig for rewards
Den sites	Hiding or sleeping	Nest box, cardboard, or cloth hammock	Security, play, climbing
Arboreal life	Climbing, foraging	Branches, ropes, platforms	Climbing, foraging, playing, exercise
Scent oriented	Smell attraction	Various scents	Exploring, exercise, rewards
Predator species	Hunting	Various small toys	Stalking, exercise
Prey species	Hiding, nocturnal	Hides, huts, coverings	Security, play, social behavior

difference and larger cages allow for greater creativity and enrichment. The size should be large enough to allow for exercise beyond a running wheel and free movement and room enough for the pet to have an elimination area or litter box when appropriate. The use of grate cage bottoms designed for feces and urine to fall through is discouraged, and plastic-bottom caging filled with appropriate substrate or bedding is more desirable. Clients should ensure cages have proper bar spacing to prevent injuries and escapes and have platforms so pets have an opportunity to be off the cage floor. Cage decorations are often species specific; but houses or hides, hammocks, beds, and thick bedding or hay will be welcome additions to toys and objects to chew. A simple way to provide enrichment is by changing the cage setup periodically. Relocating shelves and hanging ropes in different places and moving nests around allows the pet to reexplore and redecorate. Clients may offer foods in different locations to stimulate their pets to think and adapt to change and place food in places where pets have to climb to get to it.

Supervised Time-out

Because constant confinement can lead to stress and anxiety, clients should occasionally provide a safe environment outside of the cage. Allowing pets to run around and explore a larger area provides great exercise, even if just in a tiled bathroom or kitchen. Proper supervision is a must when pets are outside of their cages. Owners should ensure rooms are escape proof and ensure electric cords are inaccessible to prevent their pets from chewing on them.

Company

Safe group housing is ideal for many exotic pets, especially species that normally live in pairs or groups. With the exception of hamsters, most small mammals are happier with others of their kind; however, clients may need to be educated about such issues as sex mixing and dominance hierarchy, which may be factors with some species. In most cases, clients should not own just one of any species; but they should consult their veterinarian and breeder for advice on which sexes coexist best. Clients should also be warned of careful introduction of any new pets to existing cages to ensure safety as not all new pets are automatically accepted. Unfortunately on many occasions that someone is acquiring a new pet, the sex may be incorrectly identified by pet store employees, which can be a factor in successful cohabitation but can lead to unwanted pregnancies.

Exercise Wheels

Exercise wheels are the most common and familiar form of exercise for small mammals, and almost all rodents will use a wheel. Clients may need to be reminded that the wheel should be the right type and size for their pets to ensure that workouts are valuable. Some wheels are specifically designed for a particular species (eg, chinchillas), so be sure the one used is suitable and safe and can be cleaned.

Cardboard Boxes

Boxes are one of the cheapest and easiest ways for clients to provide their pets with an excellent source of enrichment. Almost any type of box will work, although many people think that boxes that contained food (eg, cereal) are less likely to have harmful chemicals or toxins. Some animals will make a nest in the box, and others chew or tear boxes apart. Owners can be creative and design a luxury home for pets or even build a castle from boxes.

Hiding and Nesting Places

All small mammals should have some type of hiding spot in their cage. Commercially available wooden or plastic houses work well, and other ideas include shoeboxes and baskets (**Fig. 1**). Nesting material should be provided for nesting; most pets will appreciate cut pieces of T-shirts and towels. Commercially available cotton squares also make good nest material. Most clothing is acceptable provided it has been washed, rinsed, and dried. Articles should be free of hanging strips, fringes, embroidery, sequins, and the like; material that frays easily should be avoided.

Tubes

Another easy way to enrich pets' lives is by providing tubular-shaped objects (**Fig. 2**). Most pets enjoy running through and hiding in them, and certain types of long plastic tubing are sold for ferrets particularly. Cardboard tubes from toilet paper, paper towels, or rolled carpeting are excellent options. Tubes are a must-have for most rodents, and gerbils are especially fond of chewing and shredding them.

Some species accept terracotta drainage pipes, and prairie dogs love to sleep in terra cotta flowerpots. Polyvinyl chloride pipes can be connected (pipes will fit together without glue or metal connectors) and made into a maze or hung in cages to provide beds or for exercise. They should be cleaned regularly and not hung too high. Many other safe objects, such as plastic tubing, can be found in hardware stores.

Toys

Most pet bird–style toys constructed of wood, rope, and leather are suitable for small mammals. A variety of toys can be hung in cages for pets to chew and shred. No metal objects, glass, or mirrors should be used. In all cases, common sense should be used in making proper choices. Wooden blocks, chew sticks, and other wood toys are available for small mammals. Clients can also try to satisfy their pets' chewing needs with branches of safe trees. Branches are available at pet stores, or clients can make their own as long as the wood is clean and pesticide and pest free. Most common trees (eg, elm, apple) are safe.

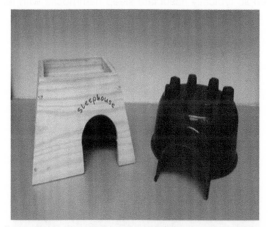

Fig. 1. Commercially available houses like these igloos (Kaytee Products Inc, Chilton, WI) and wooden houses are ideal for most small mammals and come in a variety of sizes and colors.

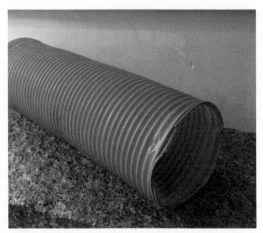

Fig. 2. These plastic tubes are ideal for play, hiding, and exercise.

Dust Baths

Dust bathing is not only for chinchillas, although they require frequent dust baths to maintain their fur coats. Many rodents will enjoy having access to a dust bath, and gerbils and degus are particular fans. Clean dust is commercially available and sold in pet stores. It can be placed in a plastic-enclosed house inside a deep box (to control the mess) and offered to the pet a few times a week.

Hiding Food

An excellent technique for enrichment is to creatively make food less readily available to pets, so they get exercise while working to find food and treats. Items can be hidden in toys, hung from the cage, or hidden in bedding (**Fig. 3**). Hiding food in hayracks or toys with special openings also provides work and exercise.

Hammocks

Although many people typically associate sleep hammocks with ferrets, other small mammals such as rats and chinchillas will also use them. Hammocks are

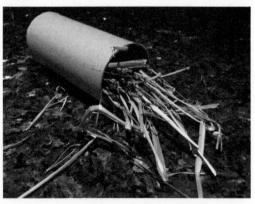

Fig. 3. Tubes are great for chewing and can be refilled with hay or other treats. Toilet paper and paper towel cardboard tubes are excellent for enrichment.

commercially available at pet stores or sold online, but pet owners can make their own from old shirts or denim pants. Cloth used for hammocks should be large and without a frayed edge, zippers, buttons, and the like. Making corner holes and using shower curtain rings is cost-effective. The leg from a pair of jeans is a great option.

SPECIES-SPECIFIC IDEAS

The following tips offer species-specific options for enrichment of pet small mammals.

Ferrets

The curious nature of ferrets and their ability to be loose in the home without fear of escape allows them to get exercise. As they age, however, ferrets sleep more and spend less time exploring and playing. Owners are advised to have more than one ferret to provide not only company for each other but also playmates. Ferrets are generally known to accept new ferrets without aggression or fighting. One issue may be introducing a young and very active ferret to an older, less-active ferret, as the younger ferret may not have the right playmate.

- Ferrets can learn to tolerate wearing a harness and may be walked on leashes near the home or in parks or other public places (except in a few cities or states where ferrets are illegal). This practice provides exercise, mental stimulation, and socialization opportunities for the ferrets and their owners.
- Most ferrets love to run through lengths of tubing. Commercially available tubing for pets or even dryer exhaust tubing or any flexible, tubelike material that is wide enough will work. Ferrets typically play when they meet in a tube. Owners can be creative with designs.
- Creating a multilevel cage in which different levels are connected by ladders and ramps provides an environment that forces ferrets to exercise.
- Filling a cardboard box with shredded paper or Styrofoam (Dow Chemical Company, Midland, MI) peanuts makes a great playpen.

Rabbits

As they age, many older rabbits tend to be less active and can become overweight. Rabbits that are not litter-box trained are often kept in cages when unsupervised, whereas some rabbits live only in small rabbit hutches without the ability to stretch and have room to exercise. Routine exercise is also thought to be an important way to help prevent gastric stasis syndrome.

- With the right yard space and setup, clients can place their rabbits in outdoor exercise pens. Most pet supply companies sell pens that confine the rabbit while still allowing it to graze and enjoy fresh air and sunshine. Owners should ensure their rabbits have access to a sheltered area and plenty of clean water. Having a reserve water bottle and bowl is advised. It is not recommended to leave them out or have them live in outside hutches.
- It is the author's recommendation that rabbits be caged at home and let out for exercise time. This practice will encourage exploring and chinning behavior; these rabbits typically do not become sedentary like free-range bunnies often do.
- Many rabbits play with toys; small stuffed animals or many types of plastic baby and toddler toys are ideal. Offer pet rabbits toys to see if they throw them around, carry them, and entertain themselves. Toys can be dangled in the cage as well.

Some dog and cat toys work well for rabbits. Chew sticks and rings are ideal, and many rabbits play by tossing or carrying them (**Fig. 4**).

- Rabbits can be clicker trained or taught to run thru mazes or obstacle courses if one commits to the training.
- Filling a cardboard box with bedding, straw, or shredded paper will allow for normal digging behavior.

Guinea Pigs

Although guinea pigs are quiet and fairly sedentary, they should still be provided with ample space. Other pigs, hide spots, and soft bedding are appreciated by these gentle pets.

- Well-socialized guinea pigs are outgoing and do not resent handling. They enjoy social time with their owners and permit brushing or petting.
- Many guinea pigs naturally exhibit rooting behaviors. Clients can encourage this behavior by hiding food and treats in clean bedding or inside certain toys.

Chinchillas

It is important to take advantage of a chinchilla's natural jumping and bouncing behaviors when designing a cage. Platforms, rope perches, and concrete bird perches work well. Some owners provide chinchillas with cholla (dried cactus; available from pet stores and pet supply companies) for chewing and climbing.

- Carpeted cat towers make great environments for chinchillas when they are out of the cage. Chinchillas should always be supervised when they are out of their cage.
- Regular dust baths are required for fur coat maintenance but also seem to be enjoyed.
- Compressed hay cubes will provide exercise, nutrition, and activity.

Rodents (Rats, Mice, Gerbils, Hamsters)

By nature most species of hamsters live a solitary existence because of territorial fighting, although some raised together may coexist with enough space. The other common pet rodents can and should live in groups with appropriate spaying and neutering.

- To enrich rodents' environments, owners can construct mazes or bury tubing under bedding.
- Many rodents can learn tricks when their owners apply positive reinforcement.

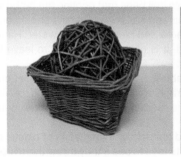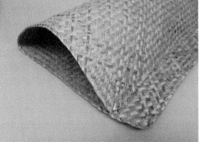

Fig. 4. Wicker and grass mats are safe for chewing, digging, and hiding food treats.

- Objects to chew and make into beds and social time are appreciated by these rodents.

Sugar Gliders

As social animals that live in colonies in the wild, gliders should never be kept alone, especially to avoid stereotypic self-destructive behaviors. Owners must give attention to their unique dietary requirements that allow for further enrichment opportunities.

- Gliders appreciate a proper running wheel.
- Pouches or hide-hammocks are a must for this species.
- Natural climbing surfaces can help keep nails short while allowing foraging sites. Sisal or avian rope perches are great additions to the cage.

Prairie Dogs

Prairie dogs tunnel, dig, and live in large colonies in the wild. A well-socialized prairie dog makes an excellent pet for those seeking a larger pet rodent.

- Cages that rest on top of large tanks are highly recommended (**Fig. 5**). The tank can be filled with bedding and hay to dig and eat, thereby allowing a more natural environment.
- Harness training allows prairie dogs to be walked in safe locations.
- Hide boxes and high perching platforms in cages.
- Prairie dogs love being petted and scratched by owners.

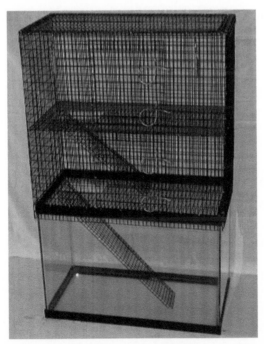

Fig. 5. Providing a cage with multiple levels connected by ramps offers pets a more stimulating environment and promotes exercise. This style is best suited for pets that would prefer deeper bedding or hay placed in the tank bottom.

SUMMARY

Veterinarians that treat small exotic mammals must consider the pets' total health not just the immediate medical needs. These concepts are foundational ideas to provide environmental enrichment, but the options are limitless. Clients can use their creativity to make ownership of pocket pets more rewarding. More importantly, they can provide a better quality of life for their special pets. The better quality of life would allow more ethical captivity conditions and prevent many psychological disorders that may develop in substandard or poorly enriched environments.

WEB SITES OF INTEREST

http://rabbit.org/shop-for-supplies/
http://www.rattoy.com/
http://www.ferret.com/toys-and-tunnels/199/
http://www.petchinchillatoys.com/
http://spoiledrottensuggies.com/
http://libbyandlouise.com/shop/product-category/small-exotic-animals/
http://www.martinscages.com/
http://www.exoticnutrition.com/

FURTHER READINGS

Bradley Bays T, Lightfoot T, Mayer J, editors. Exotic pet behavior birds, reptiles, and small mammals. St Louis (MO): Saunders Elsevier; 2006.

Church B. Enrichment for small mammals and exotic pets. Proc North Am Vet Conf 2007. p. 1640–2.

Young RJ. Environmental enrichment for captive animals. Wiley-Blackwell; 2003.

Camelid Wellness

Marty McGee Bennett, BS[a],*, Nanci L.M. Richards, DVM[b]

KEYWORDS

- New World camelid • Nutrition • Feeding plans • Shelter • Acclimation
- Body condition scoring • Enrichment • Desensitizing

KEY POINTS

- Camelid feeding management for optimal health and performance is integral to individual and herd health.
- Basic shelter from storms and inclement weather should always be provided for camelids.
- Finding the right balance in feeding camelids is critical to their health and performance, and maintaining a camelid within the ideal weight range can be managed with proper attention to nutrition and exercise.
- Camelids are shy by nature and have not been selected over their 6000 years of domestication for close contact with humans.

DIET AND NUTRITION CONSIDERATIONS

New World camelids (NWCs) are represented by 4 species: alpaca, guanaco, llama, and vicuna. The alpaca and llama are the domesticated NWC species and are the focus of this article. Although frequently classified among ruminant species, camelids are not true ruminants because they have 3 distinct stomach compartments (C-1, C-2, C-3) as opposed to the 4 distinct stomach compartments of ruminants.[1,2] However, the expanded first compartment is similar in many ways to the rumen because it is the location where the microbial fermentation of feed occurs and provides for remastication, or cud chewing.[2] As with ruminants, dietary considerations concern not only the health of the overall animal but also the health of the microbes in the first stomach compartment.[3,4] In the South American Andes, NWCs survive in the harsh environment by foraging on grasses, legumes, and forbs, and browsing on woody species, including the leaves, buds, and twigs,[5] depending on what is available to them. This behavior holds true wherever they are found.

Camelid feeding management for optimal health and performance is integral to individual and herd health. The selection of feedstuffs to meet camelid nutritional needs should

Disclosure: The authors have nothing to disclose.
[a] CAMELIDynamics, 905 Maple Street, New Smyrna Beach, FL 32169, USA; [b] Eastern Prairie Veterinary Service, PO Box 1023, St Joseph, IL 61873, USA
* Corresponding author.
E-mail address: marty@camelidynamics.com

Vet Clin Exot Anim 18 (2015) 255–280
http://dx.doi.org/10.1016/j.cvex.2015.01.006
1094-9194/15/$ – see front matter © 2015 Elsevier Inc. All rights reserved.

be based on the geography of their location, its abundances and deficiencies, as well as the management of the herd (free choice grazing vs dry lot). Each animal, and its health status, including age and intended purpose, dictates the specific nutritional requirements of that individual.[6]

A proper feeding regimen for NWC should always include a sustainable forage source, clean fresh water, and proper vitamins and minerals. Additional supplementation may be required to balance the diet or to address individual animal health conditions, as discussed later.

Forage nutritional profile measures include protein, carbohydrate, and fat content, as well as certain significant minerals (eg, calcium, phosphorus, potassium and magnesium). Hays and pastures are analyzed for nutritional components such as crude protein (CP), total digestible nutrients (TDN; a measure of energy), neutral detergent fiber (a measure of digestible fiber), and acid detergent fiber (a measure of indigestible fiber). CP and TDN are some of the most commonly used measures to determine feed quality. As found in North American hays and pastures, the estimated NWC requirements of CP and TDN are 8% to 14% and 50% to 70%, respectively. The lower values address the nutrient requirements for maintenance and the higher values are appropriate for early growth or lactation in camelids.[5]

It is typically advised to separate animals into like groups and feed them based on their individual needs, to ensure that each animal receives the proper amount and quality of nutrients. Examples of different living and feeding groups include breeding males, pregnant females, lactating females, nonreproductive females and geldings, and crias/weanlings. Also consider that weaker, thinner animals may be driven away from the food, whereas the stronger, more dominant animals may receive more than what is required for them. The following list provides a feeding approach based on certain animal groups and their specific nutrient needs. CP and TDN are frequently noted and discussed because they are often easily measured feed components from which to determine feed composition and quality.[7] They are not the only considerations, but do provide a guide from which to begin to build an appropriate diet.

ANIMAL GROUPS AND SUGGESTED FEEDING PLANS

- Lactation[6]
  - Nursing dam with cria: highest nutrient needs; high-quality forage plus supplementation, including minerals and vitamins as appropriate
  - From 12% to 14% CP, 60% to 70% TDN
- Growth[6]
  - Weanlings up to 1.5 years: highest nutrient needs; high-quality forage plus supplementation, including minerals and vitamins as appropriate
  - From 14% to 16% CP, 55% to 65% TDN
- Maintenance[6]
  - Males older than 1 year: low nutrient needs, unless working/actively breeding (adjust accordingly); low-quality to moderate-quality forage
  - Pregnant females in months 1 to 8: low nutrient needs, maintain body condition; low-quality to moderate-quality forage plus protein, minerals, and vitamins as appropriate
  - Breeding females: low nutrient needs, maintain body condition (not overweight or loss of proper condition); low-quality to moderate-quality forage, minerals and vitamins as appropriate
  - From 8% to 10% CP, 50% to 55% TDN (up to 60% TDN for breeding males)

- Late pregnancy[6]
  - Pregnant females in months 9 to 11: moderate-quality to high-quality forage plus mineral and vitamin supplementation
  - From 10% to 12% CP, 55% to 70% TDN
- Submaintenance[6]
  - Obese animals: lowest nutrient needs; low-quality forage plus mineral and vitamin supplement only (unless pregnant, then feed as described earlier)
  - From 8% to 9% CP, 45% to 33% TDN

Again, fresh, clean water is a vital component of proper camelid nutrition and should always be provided, along with the previously discussed feeds.

Supplementation (grain, pelleted feed) is often incorporated into camelid diets outside South America.[5] Commercial supplements are available that are specifically formulated for camelids. However, as noted in the feeding regimens listed previously, all camelids do not require this type of supplementation.

In situations in which hay or supplements are fed, space is an important consideration with camelids to ensure that each animal gets an appropriate amount. Crowding creates competition, so more space is better. Providing multiple feeding stations is helpful.

Minerals are an important inclusion in the NWC diet as well. Knowledge of what the diet is providing and the geographic deficiencies and excesses should be considered. There are species-specific commercially prepared loose mineral blends available that address general needs. They can be offered free choice or top dressed at a specific rate (grams per day). Free-choice white salt (NaCl) should also be available for NWCs.[5]

It has been documented that heavily fibered animals may experience seasonal vitamin D deficiencies.[8] Of particular concern are crias born in the fall months in the northern hemisphere, and even other times of the year when camelids are located in areas where cloudy conditions may persist (eg, Pacific Northwest). Supplementation with products containing vitamin D_3 (injectables or paste) has been suggested. Care must be taken in the dosing amount and frequency because toxicities can occur.

As with other nutrients, it is important to consider the geography where the animals are kept, and the surpluses or deficiencies therein, to address camelids' mineral requirements. Selenium is one such element. In some areas soils are deficient in selenium and supplementation with oral or injectable minerals is recommended. In other geographic locations selenium can reach toxic levels through feeding certain grass hays.[9]

In addition, NWCs are similarly sensitive to copper, as are sheep, and attention must be paid to the copper content of feeds, minerals, or other supplements that may be fed or administered.[9]

HOUSING AND SHELTER

Basic shelter from storms and inclement weather should be provided. Housing provided can vary from a basic run-in shed (3-sided) structure to an enclosed barn with or without stalls (**Figs. 1** and **2**). Camelids are highly visual and seem to prefer a less closed-in environment, thus keeping their ability to identify threats intact. It is not surprising to find them staying outside rather than going into a barn, even during weather events. In general, porches attached to a barn are more desirable and more fully used than the inside of the barn. Shelter should also provide critical shade in hotter temperatures as well as the more obvious protection from rain, ice, and snow (**Fig. 3**). Providing proper ventilation is also important to the animals' health and well-being. In hot climates fans are helpful for insect control and cooling.

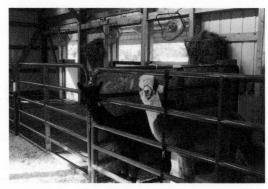

Fig. 1. Simple barn with panels used as dividers. (*Courtesy of* April Polansky (photographer) and Fallengrund Alpacas, Butler, IL.)

Predator concerns can be addressed by providing a small pasture that is secure with high fencing and an electrified wire at the top and bottom adjoining a barn or porch, rather than closing animals in a barn at night or when left unattended.

See **Figs. 1–3** for examples of different types of housing for NWCs.

Feeders and Feeding

In their native land, llamas and alpacas forage widely to get enough to eat and therefore do not naturally compete for food. In view of this, feeding arrangements that require animals to eat in close contact cause stress and might prevent some animals from having access to adequate amounts of food. More feeder space is best and feeding at least some of their diet of hay on the ground outside in the pasture under the shelter of trees offers exercise, reduces competition, and provides a more

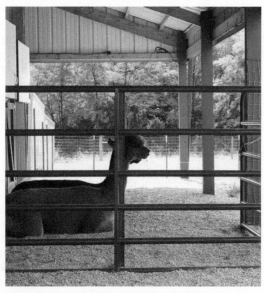

Fig. 2. Porches are the preferred loafing spot for camelids. (*Courtesy of* April Polansky (photographer) and Fallengrund Alpacas, Butler, IL.)

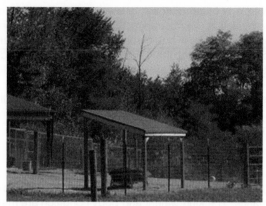

Fig. 3. Simple shade shelters for hotter summertime temperatures. (*Courtesy of* April Polan-sky (photographer) and Fallengrund Alpacas, Butler, IL.)

enriched environment. If animals must be fed in close proximity, using panels to create barriers between feeders can help reduce competition (**Fig. 4**).

SUBSTRATE

Camelids frequently lie in a sternal position, also known as kushing, and need proper surfaces to kush on. Therefore, if concrete is the flooring available, additional padding or bedding is recommended to reduce stress on the body, whether kushing, standing, or walking about. Rubber mats, straw, and similar substrates are appropriate. Wood shavings are not recommended because they contaminate the fiber and are difficult to remove. A sand substrate that can be soaked with water in the summer helps with cooling.

TEMPERATURE AND ENVIRONMENT

Camelids can live and thrive in a variety of climates and temperature ranges, but consideration should be given to their comfort for optimal health and peak perfor-mance. Provisions should be made not only for keeping the animals dry and warm in the winter but also to provide air movement or cooling in the summer.

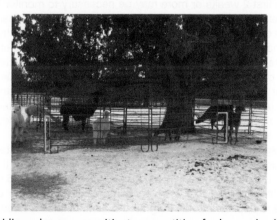

Fig. 4. Panels dividing a larger area mitigate competition for hay and pellets.

The appropriate timing of fiber removal, or shearing, is one method of temperature control and thermoregulation. As fiber animals, shearing is done to harvest the fiber, but is also provides body cooling in hot, humid conditions. Shearing should take place in moderate temperatures so that the animals have a chance to acclimate before extreme temperature swings, while allowing them to grow a full fleece before the following winter.

Also to be considered is that very young, very old, small, or infirm animals may require additional warmth to maintain an appropriate body temperature. The local climate dictates the management required.

IDEAL WEIGHT

As previously discussed, finding the right balance in feeding camelids is critical to their health and performance. Tracking weight and body condition are measurements that help in assessing the animal. These parameters can serve as indicators of the overall health of the camelid.

Typical adult weights of the NWCs[10]:

- Alpaca: 55 to 90 kg
- Guanaco: 100 to 120 kg
- Llama: 113 to 250 kg
- Vicuna: 45 to 55 kg

Typical birth weights of NWC[10]:

- Alpaca: 6 to 9 kg
- Guanaco: 8 to 15 kg
- Llama: 8 to 18 kg
- Vicuna: 4 to 6 kg

Maintaining a camelid within the ideal weight range can be managed with proper attention to nutrition and exercise. Both extremes, being too thin and carrying excess weight, are detrimental to the animal's life expectancy, fiber production, and reproductive capabilities (eg, fertility, lactation).[11]

It is recommended that camelids be weighed regularly and have their body condition score (BCS) assessed. For adults, if the animal appears otherwise healthy, this can be done monthly. For crias, particularly neonates, weight checks daily or every other day for the first 2 weeks or more may be necessary to monitor for appropriate growth and development and measure the mothers' lactation capabilities to meet the energy needs of the young crias. As long as the cria appears healthy, appropriately active, and well nourished, biweekly or even monthly weight checks until the cria reaches approximately 22 to 27 kg in body weight is typically adequate. At that point, weights can be coordinated with typical herd health checks. Scales are available that work well for camelids, but any scale that is safe, for humans and animals, and large enough to get an accurate weight, will work. Creating a system for weighing that does not involve haltering animals makes short work of the process and is easier and safer for the animals (**Figs. 5** and **6**A).

In addition to regular weighing, the BCS is a subjective grading system that requires feeling the animals by hand, to assess the subcutaneous fat mass of the animal. From this assessment, a number score is given on a scale of either 1 to 5 (which often includes increments of 0.5) or 1 to 9 (1 = very thin/emaciated; 5 or 9 = obese).[12] Using either BCS scale is appropriate, as long as the denominator is known and remains constant.

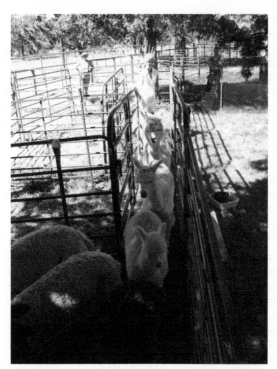

Fig. 5. Training the animals to walk through the narrow lane and over a rubber mat.

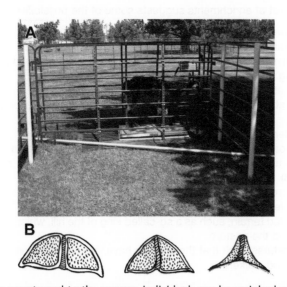

Fig. 6. (*A*) Once accustomed to the process, individuals can be weighed without the need for haltering or leading. (*B*) Lumber region assessment of BCS (*left to right*): obese (BCS, 5 out of 5 or 9 out of 9); moderate weight (BCS, 3 out of 5 or 5 out of 9); very thin/emaciated (BCS, 1 out of 5 or 1 out of 9). (*Courtesy of* Stephen R. Purdy, DVM, Nunoa Project and North American Camelid Studies Program, Amherst, MA; with permission.)

The primary location to begin the BCS assessment is over the lumber region of the animal (behind the ribs and in front of the hips). To do this, gently hold the animal by placing a hand with the webbed area between the thumb and the index finger snug along the backbone of the animal across the lumber region to feel the soft tissue mass compared with the prominence of the vertebral spinous process.[12] Once a score has been determined, also compare with the prominence and fat covering the ribs and the fat mass between the hind and front legs to make minor adjustments to the score, if needed (usually no more than 0.5–1.0 score adjustment, in either direction). **Fig. 6**B shows high, medium, and low ranges of the BCS, across the lumbar region, and may help in making the assessment.

To be effective, these measurements (weight and BCS) should be recorded to track an individual camelid's overall health. Trends or changes noted in the animal may help to identify problems or disease processes that should be addressed.

ENVIRONMENTAL ENRICHMENT

Paddock size is not as important as the availability of interesting and plentiful low-calorie forage and browse. Variation in the environment, such as the availability of hills, trees, roadside activity, and conspecifics, are more important than the size of the paddock. Although camelids get along well with other kinds of barnyard livestock they prefer the company of other camelids of the same species. A single llama or alpaca should never be kept alone without other camelids. Ideally llamas have other llamas and alpacas have other alpacas; however, sole llamas or alpacas accommodate to life with the other camelid species. Mixed herds of both species also work well and can be managed easily together. Camelids spend a lot of time eating but they also have a rich behavioral palette and the more enrichment opportunities you offer the more you see.

The following list of enrichments suggests some of the possibilities[1]:

- Create browse by offering limbs
- Provide rotational grazing access to new areas periodically
- Offer hay in multiple locations outside requiring foraging behaviors when weather permits (**Fig. 7**)
- Offer a variety of hays
- Offer oat straw to extend the amount of time animals spend eating and ruminating
- Offer smaller amounts of hay more frequently
- Vary the location and method of offering hay, grains, and treats
- Provide scratching posts, street sweeper brushes, or brushes mounted on the wall (**Fig. 8**)
- Provide mirrors (**Fig. 9**)
- Add water features (eg, sprinklers, wading pools for summer)
- Provide varied terrain, such as a so-called king of the hill, which is easily created with fill dirt in the pasture
- Arrange pastures such that the animals have things to observe, such as traffic, bicyclists, and walkers

---

[1] When adding dietary elements as enrichment, take care to consider the diet in total and make any changes gradually. The nutritional information provided earlier in this article should be considered the central part of a camelid diet. Regular weighing and body condition scoring provides the information needed to make sure that a diet is providing the appropriate nutrition.

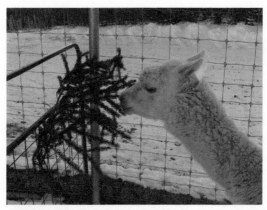

Fig. 7. Spruce tree branches are a particular favorite.

MENTAL STIMULATION

Camelids require knowledge and skill to be caught, haltered, and led in a way that is palatable (discussed later); however, off-lead training using an event marker (clicker) and toys are universally met with enthusiasm. The following ideas represent some of the possibilities:

- A treat panel with holes covered by small, movable doors secured with 1 screw provides an interesting place to hide carrots. The animals will learn to move the panel aside to gain access to the treat (**Fig. 10**).

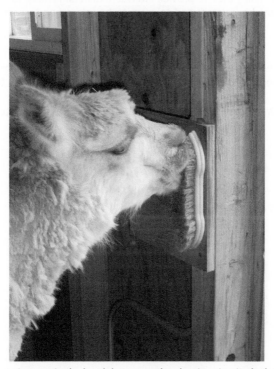

Fig. 8. Carrots create interest in the brush but, once they begin using it, the brush is reinforcing.

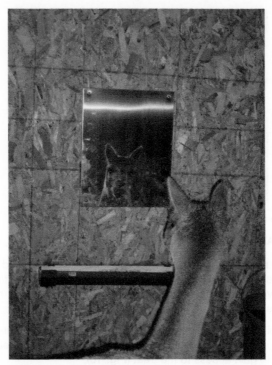

Fig. 9. Mirrors have many uses: to provide interest in mineral feeders, to offer company for an animal that must be isolated, and to seem to be interesting to camelids (similarly to mirrors for birds).

- Little bowls with holes drilled in the middle and mounted on a dowel secured to a ledge creating the wobbly dish toy. Treats are placed between the small dishes (**Fig. 11**).
- Plastic jars with holes make carrot roll-arounds, similar to a buster cube for dogs (**Fig. 12**).

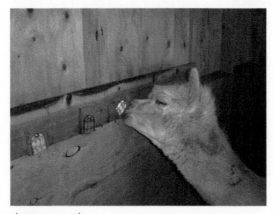

Fig. 10. A homemade treat panel.

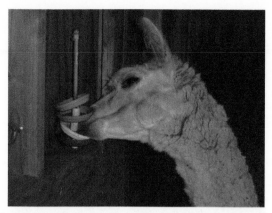

Fig. 11. Treats between the dishes provide interest and a challenge.

- In the wintertime, caching food in snow holes or at the far edges of the pasture can provide additional opportunities for foraging, investigating their environment, and for exercise. This searching appeals to their seeking instincts and desire to search for food (**Fig. 13**).
- Clicker training is remarkably efficient and fun. Given that clicker training is positive reinforcement based, it has the added benefit of ensuring that the animal is a willing participant. Off-lead work is an effective way to increase the level of trust between human and camelid. Target training is both fun and useful in herd management and training. The imagination is the only limiting factor. Mazes, jumps, weaving between poles, walking through hoops, standing and sitting on rugs, walking through a tunnel, and ringing a bell are all activities that camelids enjoy (**Fig. 14**).

Getting camelids to try new things often involves food. Grain works, but carrots, grapes, and garden vegetable treats are preferable to too much grain or other sugary treats. Just because a camelid will eat something does not mean that it should be used for enrichment. Make sure that healthy foods are being offered. If camelids do not know about healthy treats, it can be a challenge to get them to try a new food. Here are a few ideas:

- Cut the new food up into very small pieces that are easily chewed
- Introduce the food to a grain treat that your animals already like

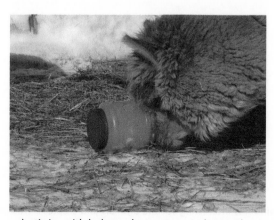

Fig. 12. Carrots in a plastic jar with holes make treats more interesting and they last longer.

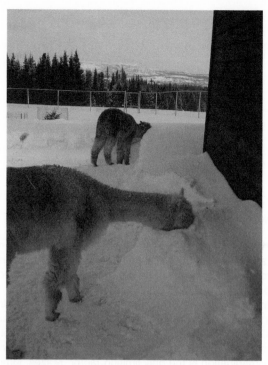

Fig. 13. Hiding food in snow or small caches of particularly good hay around the pasture keeps the animals foraging.

- Mixing shredded carrots in with alfalfa leaves can encourage the animals to acquire the taste, because it is difficult to separate the small bits of carrots from the leaves
- Be persistent

BEHAVIOR TRAINING FOR HEALTHY INTERACTION WITH OWNERS

Camelids are shy by nature and have not been selected in their 6000 years of domestication for close contact with humans. A camelid's long neck provides the handler a

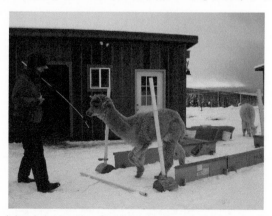

Fig. 14. Clicker training is interesting for the animals and creates a trusting relationship in addition to teaching useful behaviors.

significant and potentially dangerous amount of leverage. Coupled with a small head, this leverage provides a significant challenge when it comes to haltering and leading (**Fig. 15**). For positive interactions with camelids it is necessary to spend some time desensitizing the animal to human approach and proximity.

Handling Area Setup

Using laneways leading to a smaller paddock and ultimately to a catch pen (no larger than 3 × 3 m [10 × 10 feet] square and 1.2–1.5 m [4–5 feet] in height) makes catching easier and more palatable for the animals (**Fig. 16**). Calling the animals in for a food treat is a good initial plan but a well-designed system that allows handlers to move animals to a confined area with herding tools is crucial for good management. The use of 1.2-m(4 foot) herding poles allows handlers to communicate with camelids from a distance, which is easier and safer for the animals (**Fig. 17**). Tying a rope or using a nylon tape attached to the corner of a paddock allows handlers to create a temporary fence or laneway leading to a smaller area (**Fig. 18**). Ropes or herding tape is not suitable for trapping animals in a corner. Herding tape is only useful for creating a temporary path to a safe handling area.

A handling area with pens of various sizes, including 2.7 × 2.7 m (9 × 9 feet) and 1.2 to 1.5 m high (4–5 feet), which is useful for catching, haltering, restraint-free injection, and other management tasks; 2.7 × 0.9 m (9 × 3 feet), which is useful for trimming toenails; and 2.7 × 8.2 m (9 × 27 feet), which is useful for initial lead training, allows handlers to work with containment instead of using restraint (**Fig. 19**). Owners who do not have a proper setup but who own trailers can use a trailer as a handling area. Parking

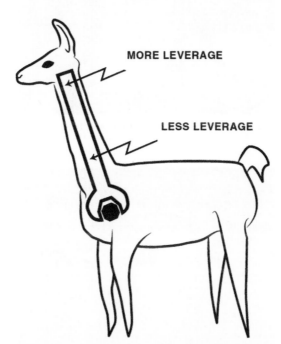

MORE LEVERAGE

LESS LEVERAGE

Fig. 15. The further away the head is from the center of mass the more leverage control of the head offers the handler. It is important to use this additional leverage responsibly. (*From* Bennett M. The camelid companion. New Smyrna Beach (FL): Raccoon Press; 2001. p. 93; with permission.)

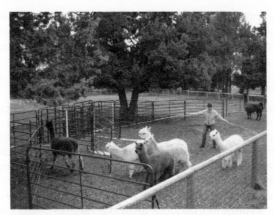

Fig. 16. An intermediately sized handling area adjacent to a small pen for catching allows force-free catching and handling.

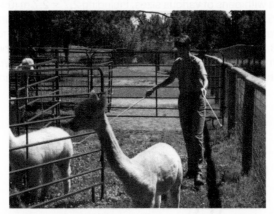

Fig. 17. Sorting animals with wands is more efficient and feels safer for the animals.

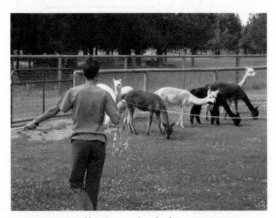

Fig. 18. Herding tape or rope is effective and safe for creating a temporary fence line but should never be used to trap animals in a corner.

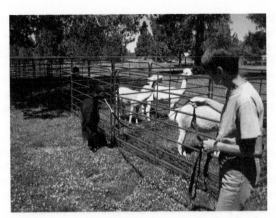

Fig. 19. Teaching animals to lead in a long narrow container with a long lead means that the handler never needs to hold tightly to the animal's head causing the animal to kush, buck, or rear and risking potential injury.

the trailer at the end of a laneway and herding the animals into the trailer is easily done (**Fig. 20**). Once confined to the trailer, management and husbandry tasks are more easily accomplished.

Camelids react adversely to restraint and often fight and hurt both themselves and the handler when held or tied; conversely, using a small, secure working area or crowding

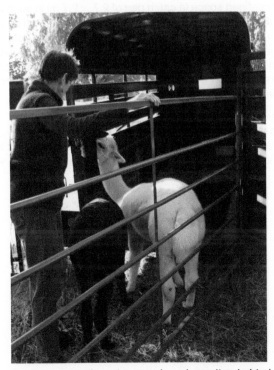

Fig. 20. Herding animals into a trailer using panels and standing behind the group of animals is a safe, easy way to load animals that have not been taught to lead.

animals together in a small area facilitates safe herd management (**Fig. 21**). When feeding, cleaning up, or visiting the paddock it is best for handlers to keep their hands to themselves and avoid the tendency to reach out and touch the animals. Likewise, greet the camelids with the back of your hand or your nose when they come over to investigate you (**Fig. 22**). Nothing is more important to a camelid than the ability to run from perceived danger, therefore providing a clear escape route relative to any walls, fences, or pens helps greatly to create an enhanced feeling of safety in their environment.

Desensitizing a Camelid to Human Approach

The camelid industry evolved with a system of catching that involves trapping the animal in a corner, approaching with arms outstretched and holding the animal by the neck and wrestling the animal until it stopped resisting. This approach, known as flooding or response blocking, with respect to human approach is dangerous for both animal and handler and creates fear and distrust. If you are working with a camelid that has been cornered and grabbed in the past you need to desensitize the animal to your approach before you can halter the animal without force or develop a fear-free relationship. Systematic desensitization to a human's approach or the presentation of a stimulus in the smallest possible increments so that the animal can accept each increment without fear is a better system with several positive outcomes. A 1.2-m (4-foot) wand with a clip attached to the end as a way of passing a catch rope of 3.4 to 3.7 m (11–12 feet) over the top of the head and around the neck is recommended. This system allows the handler to break down catching an animal into smaller increments and replaces a fearful response with acceptance.

The success of this method requires the handler to learn how to stand behind the animal's eye in a confined space (a catch pen of 2.7 × 2.7 m) in such a way as to offer an escape route (**Fig. 23**) along with learning to maintain a neutral connection through the rope around the neck (**Fig. 24**). A wand and rope in a proper catch pen is the most efficient way to desensitize a camelid to your approach. It may be helpful to desensitize the animal to the wand by moving the wand slowly back and forth over the animal's head before attaching the rope to the wand. The following are some hints for using a wand effectively:

- Make sure you are providing an escape route.
- The wand goes from the back to the front of the animal. Putting the wand in front of the animal in an attempt to put it over from the front to the back closes the escape route with the wand, creates fear, and defeats the purpose of using the wand (**Fig. 25**).

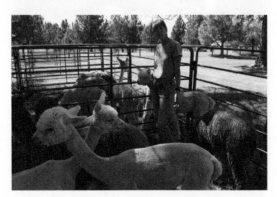

Fig. 21. Packing a pen is safer than working with animals alone. A well-packed pen means that there is approximately 20% to 25% of space unoccupied by animals.

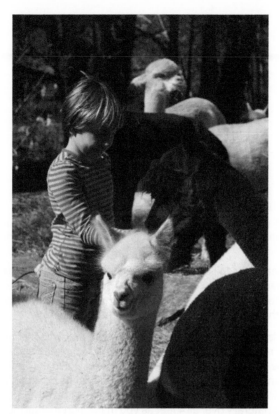

Fig. 22. A polite greeting by both the child and the animal; nonthreatening from both points of view.

- Keep the wand low; it should only be above head level for a second or two.
- Use the full length of the wand; remember that the purpose of the wand is to keep you far enough away from the animal that it feels out of danger (outside arm's length; **Fig. 26**).

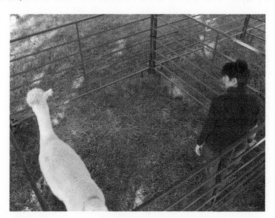

Fig. 23. A handler can offer an escape route even when the animal is in a small area by remaining in a position behind the animal's eye.

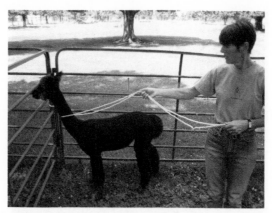

Fig. 24. A neutral connection means that the handler can quickly influence an animal's balance with a signal on the line but there is no steady tension in the line.

- When you reach out initially with the wand, keep it in place behind the neck; do not withdraw and reach out repeatedly. The animal is likely to move into the escape route when you reach out with the wand. Keep the wand in place and make sure that you continue to provide an escape route.

Once the rope is around the animal's neck, the wand is disconnected, and you have both ends of the rope in your hands, make sure that you keep slack in the rope and remain behind the eye offering a forward escape route within the confines of the catch pen (**Fig. 27**). Using the rope to hold the animal against its will is only marginally less frightening. The idea is to use the rope to communicate with and help the animal remain in balance naturally over all 4 feet as you make incremental movements toward the animal. The process is like a conversation in which you ask with your body, "Do you feel safe if I move this close?" If the animal remains standing, its answer is "Yes." If it begins to shift its balance in preparation to take a step, the answer is "No." The response should be to shift the animal's balance back to a neutral stance with a quick, short signal on the rope followed by a release of tension, and at the same time move away from the animal. This movement indicates that you will back off to provide safety when the animal feels threatened. This process is often skipped

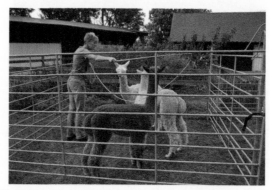

Fig. 25. The wand is held as low as possible and is only above the head for a second or two. The idea is to use the wand to catch the animal slowly and deliberately.

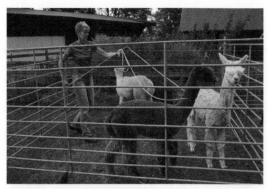

Fig. 26. The purpose of the wand is to keep the handler away from the animal so as not to frighten the animal. The wand is used to bring the rope back to the handler.

in favor of the more expedient corner grab hold approach; however, an animal that is not desensitized to human approach must be restrained for even the simplest handling and will never trust its human caretakers (**Fig. 28**).

Halter Fit

In my experience, improper halter fit and its related effects create a significant impact on the well-being of camelids. The following are specific outcomes associated with halter fit:

- Most camelids misbehave when on a lead rope because their halters do not fit
- Most difficult-to-halter camelids are that way because of early experiences with the halter; both its fit and the way it is introduced
- When a llama or alpaca is wearing a halter with an improper fit it is more difficult to handle; this means that shearing, trimming toenails, giving injections, or doing ultrasonography or any other medical procedure can all be adversely affected by improper halter fit

A camelid's small head is carried at a right angle to the neck, and the leverage provided by the long neck makes proper halter fit more difficult and much more important than it is with other barnyard animals that are typically haltered (see **Fig. 15**).[13–15] Llamas, and to a larger degree alpacas, have much shorter nose bones than might be expected (**Fig. 29**). Most of what is often called the nose is cartilage not bone.

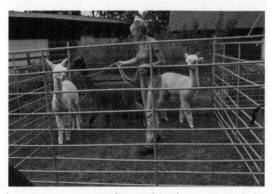

Fig. 27. Maintain the escape route even after catching by remaining behind the animal's eye.

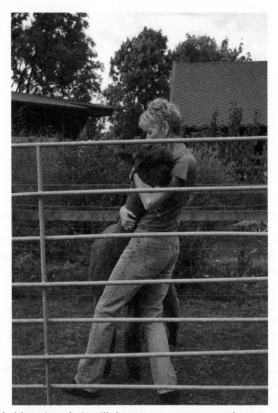

Fig. 28. Animals held against their will do not get near or trust humans.

The nose bone on most adult camelids ends approximately an inch in front of the eyes and provides little solid bone on which to hang a halter nose band.

Most people have trouble fitting a halter because they do not understand camelid anatomy and its effect on halter fitting.[13–15] Camelids are semiobligate nasal

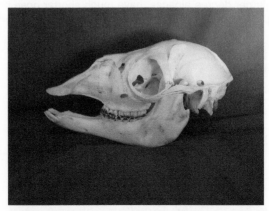

Fig. 29. The nose bone is short even on an adult. Haltering and leading young camelids must be done with great care and skill.

breathers, so they breathe largely, but not entirely, through their noses. A camelid can die if its nasal passages are completely blocked. Because of this anatomy, any suggestion that the halter may slip forward and off the nose bone is going to frighten the animal and potentially create a serious panic reaction. In order for the halter to be both safe and comfortable the halter must fit around the head with the crown piece up high and snug just behind the ears and the throat piece contacting the back third of the jaw bone (**Fig. 30**). The nose band must be large enough to provide room for the animal to yawn, take in grass and grain, and ruminate without restriction. However, there are many halters available that do not fit properly no matter how they are adjusted. A well-proportioned and well-designed halter includes:

- Adjustments in the nose band and crown piece
- Many holes on both the nose band and crown piece that are close together (~6 mm apart), offering a wide range of adjustments
- A nose band that is large enough to fit comfortably (a finger or two of slack) well up on the nose bone just in front of the eye; the part of the halter that contacts the jawbone (the throat latch) should contact the jawbone on the heaviest part of the jaw bone about two-thirds of the way rearward of the front teeth (**Figs. 31–33**).

Note that it is absolutely inappropriate to cover the airway of a camelid. Covering a camelid's nose and mouth with a spit mask or sock or covering the head during shearing or an unpleasant medical procedure compromises the airway, increases the animal's level of discomfort, and creates panic. Inhalation pneumonia is also possible when covering the nose and mouth. If spitting is an issue, once an animal is caught (a prerequisite for covering the airway) it is easy to aim the nose away from people, making the act of covering the airway unnecessary. Spit washes off, but bad experiences stay with an animal for a long time.

INTERACTING APPROPRIATELY WITH YOUNG CAMELIDS

Baby llamas (8–18 kg at birth) and alpacas (6–9 kg at birth) are adorable and it is difficult to imagine that they could grow up to be dangerous to humans. However, this happens all too often. Breeders with inadequate experience may make the mistake of encouraging behavior such as failure to maintain appropriate distance, physical pushing for food,

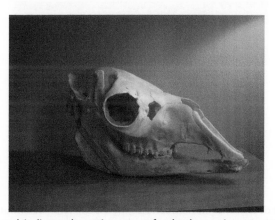

Fig. 30. The blue mark indicates the optimum area for the throat piece to contact the jaw bone.

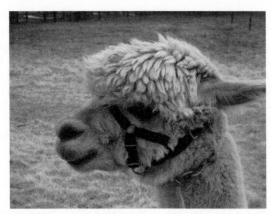

Fig. 31. This halter fits. The nose band is well up on the nose bone and the throat piece contacts the last third of the jaw bone.

rearing, and jumping, which may be tolerated in a young animal but later turns into dangerous behavior in an animal weighing 70 to 200 kg (**Fig. 34**).[13–15]

Although this behavior is more problematic and more common in males given their tendency to be territorial and more physical with each other, females that are not raised to be aware of their size and proximity to humans can develop the same problematic behaviors. Bottle-feeding a youngster might be fun to contemplate but it is time consuming, difficult, and often leads to inappropriate behavior directed at humans. When possible, bottle babies should remain in the herd and be fed from a bottle hanger in a small creep area, with little or no contact with humans during feeding times (**Fig. 35**). Young animals should not be picked up, held, cuddled, wrestled with, encouraged to sit on the lap of a human, or encouraged to stand too close to or follow humans. In short, these animals should not be treated like a family dog. Young children should always be supervised when interacting with animals and camelids are no different. Wrestling with or physically playing with young camelids puts both the child and the camelid at risk.

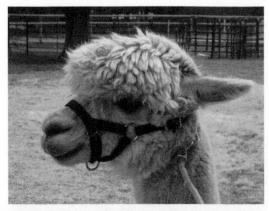

Fig. 32. This halter does not fit. The nose band is tying the animal's mouth shut. The throat piece is well forward on the jaw bone, compromising the ability of the animal to use the jaw to eat.

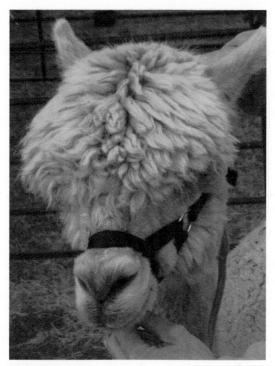

Fig. 33. The nose band will compress the soft cartilage when any downward pressure is applied, compromising the airway.

BEHAVIOR TRAINING FOR HEALTHY INTERACTION WITH CONSPECIFICS

With enough to eat, feeders set well apart, and an interesting environment, most females get along most of the time. Geldings housed with females are usually the last to eat and are often alone or relegated to a nanny role with youngsters. For this reason multiple geldings in a group of females are usually more content.

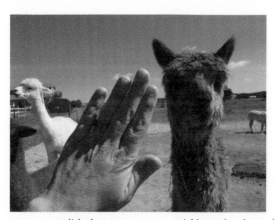

Fig. 34. Precocious young camelids that come up too quickly or closely can learn to stay back.

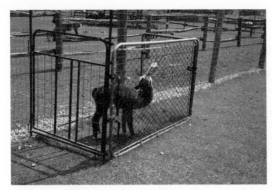

Fig. 35. A small area that the cria can enter and feed from a bottle on a hanger prevents confusing interactions with humans.

Only the finest males should be considered for breeding. Nonbreeding males are more content and easier to house and manage if they are gelded. If maintenance of a group of intact males is important, it is recommended that the fighting teeth be removed at approximately 2 to 3 years of age. There are a total of 6 fighting teeth: 4 on the top and 2 on the bottom. They are sharp and angled caudally and are dangerous to other males and humans (**Fig. 36**). These teeth should be significantly trimmed under sedation with a grinding tool (such as a Dremel) or dental saw by a qualified veterinarian. They require repeat management every 1 to 2 years, even in gelded males. In addition, care should be taken in groups of males that all animals in the group have access to water, food, and shade. Often a particular male blocks the access to resources, and this can be prevented with additional feeding stations, water buckets, and sheds. Intact males fight less if they are kept in an area without visual contact with females. In some cases it is not possible to keep an intact male with other males without risk to the group; however, this is not the norm and a certain amount of spitting, wrestling, and loud vocalizations are normal and should not be considered reason to house males alone (**Fig. 37**).

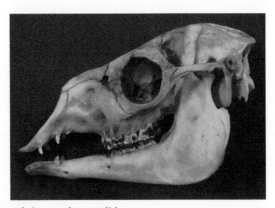

Fig. 36. Fighting teeth in a male camelid.

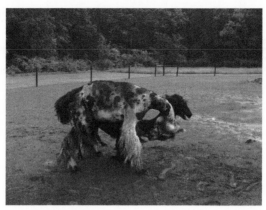

Fig. 37. Males fight and make some noise doing it. It is good exercise and normal.

REFERENCES

1. Fowler ME. Digestive system. In: Fowler ME, editor. Medicine and surgery of camelids. 3rd edition. Ames (IA): Wiley-Blackwell; 2010. p. 364–5.
2. Van Saun RJ. Nutritional requirements and assessing nutritional status in camelids. Vet Clin North Am Food Anim Pract 2009;25(2):265–79.
3. House JK, Gunn AA. Manifestations and management of disease in neonatal ruminants. In: Smith BP, editor. Large animal internal medicine. 4th edition. St Louis (MO): Mosby Elsevier; 2009. p. 368.
4. McSweeney C, Mackie R. Background study paper 61: micro-organisms and ruminant digestion: state of knowledge, trends and future prospects. FAO Document Repository. FAO Commission on Genetic Resources for Food and Agriculture; 2012. Accessed October 14, 2014.
5. Van Saun RJ. Feeds for camelids. In: Cebra C, Anderson DE, Tibary A, et al, editors. Llama and alpaca care; medicine, surgery, reproduction, nutrition, and herd health. St Louis (MO): Saunders; 2013. p. 80–91.
6. Van Saun RJ. Feeding management systems. In: Cebra C, Anderson DE, Tibary A, et al, editors. Llama and alpaca care; medicine, surgery, reproduction, nutrition, and herd health. St Louis (MO): Saunders; 2013. p. 91–100.
7. Smith BB, Timm KI, Long PO. Llama and alpaca neonatal care. Corvallis (OR): Bixby Press; 1996. p. 37.
8. Parker JE, Timm KI, Smith BB, et al. Seasonal interaction in serum vitamin D concentration and bone density in alpacas. Am J Vet Res 2002;63(7): 948–53.
9. Van Saun RJ, Cebra C. Nutritional diseases. In: Cebra C, Anderson DE, Tibary A, et al, editors. Llama and alpaca care; medicine, surgery, reproduction, nutrition, and herd health. St Louis (MO): Saunders; 2013. p. 121–39.
10. Fowler ME. General biology and evolution. In: Medicine and surgery of camelids. 3rd edition. Ames (IA): Wiley-Blackwell; 2010. p. 14.
11. Maas J, Stratton-Phelps M. Alterations in body weight or size. In: Smith BP, editor. Large animal internal medicine. 4th edition. St Louis (MO): Mosby Elsevier; 2009. p. 147–69.
12. Van Saun RJ, Herdt T. Nutritional assessment. In: Cebra C, Anderson DE, Tibary A, et al, editors. Llama and alpaca care; medicine, surgery,

reproduction, nutrition, and herd health. St Louis (MO): Saunders; 2013. p. 100–23.
13. Bennett M. The camelid companion.
14. Bennett M. Available at: www.camelidynamics.com.
15. Bennett M. Available at: www.camelidynamics.com/forums. Articles and posts on the interactive online forum.

Reptile Wellness Management

Stacey Leonatti Wilkinson, DVM, DABVP (Reptile and Amphibian)

KEYWORDS

• Reptile • Husbandry • Nutrition • Enrichment • Training

KEY POINTS

• Proper husbandry is the most important factor in keeping reptiles healthy. Deficiencies in husbandry lead to stress and disease.

• Larger, more naturalistic enclosures are recommended in order to decrease stress and encourage more natural behaviors.

• Enrichment programs for reptiles encourage mental stimulation, foraging, and exercise, all of which can benefit their overall health and welfare.

• Operant conditioning and desensitization can be used to train reptiles, shaping behaviors that allow the keeper to interact with the animal in a less stressful manner.

Reptiles have been kept in captivity for many years, and knowledge of their care is always evolving and improving. Proper husbandry is the most important factor in keeping captive reptiles healthy. The number one cause of illness in captive reptiles, and their subsequent presentation to the reptile veterinarian, is improper husbandry. Nutrition, caging, temperature, lighting, humidity, substrate, and so forth are all important for a captive reptile's health. In more recent years, concern over providing exercise and opportunities to exhibit natural behaviors has also increased. These changes allow an animal to act more like a wild conspecific, resulting in a leaner condition, more successful breeding, and longer lifespans.[1] Reptiles that lack appropriate temperature zones, lighting, humidity, hiding places, and proper nutrition are more susceptible to disease than those that are kept under appropriate conditions.[1] Captivity itself creates stress, as an enclosure would almost never be the same size as an animal's normal home range.[2] Improper husbandry conditions commonly create stress, as do constant changes (changing substrate, cages, accessories, adding cage mates), excessive handling, or placing the cage in a high-traffic area.[1–3] The stress response causes immunosuppression leading to increased incidence of disease.[1–4] It can also cause changes in behavior related to reproduction and can even inhibit estrogen and the

There is no conflict of interest to report.
Department of Clinical Sciences, Avian and Exotic Animal Care, North Carolina State University College of Veterinary Medicine, 8711 Fidelity Boulevard, Raleigh, NC 27617, USA
E-mail address: yecats_2@hotmail.com

production of vitellogenin in females and decrease testosterone concentrations in males.[2,4] Knowing what is necessary for a species is needed to prevent problems.

There are more than 7000 species of reptiles. Species vary widely in terms of diet, natural behaviors, environment, and so forth; their captive care requirements vary just as widely. It is impossible for one to learn about all species, but there are general guidelines for the care of the different orders and families of reptiles. The animal's natural history should be researched and its care made to mimic that as much as possible. It is prudent for the reptile veterinarian to learn proper husbandry for the common species he or she will be treating and to learn about the products available for reptile owners to purchase. It is also helpful to compile a list of books and Web sites available for reptile owners to refer to for proper husbandry information and to find information about an uncommonly kept species he or she is being asked to treat. Some of these resources are listed in **Table 1**. With the advent of the Internet, there is a wealth of information available; one must learn how to separate the good information from the bad.

NUTRITION

Proper nutrition of captive reptiles is an area that has gone through many changes over the years and is still constantly evolving. Reptiles are ectothermic, meaning their body temperature varies with the environmental temperature; proper temperature is extremely important for proper digestion and metabolism.[3,5,6] Metabolic rates depend on the species but, in general, are approximately 65% to 75% less than the metabolic rates of mammals.[5,6] Proper husbandry is also important, as animals that are stressed or sick will not eat as readily as they should, leading to further problems. Nutritional recommendations are based on an animal's natural diet and environment, age, activity, reproductive status, season, and overall health.[3,5,7] Generally reptiles are fed more when growing, reproducing, and when active.[7] Many reptile species are able to fast for weeks to months in the wild as an adaptation for times of drought, lack of food,

Table 1 Reliable sources for husbandry information	
www.anapsid.org	Main focus is green iguanas but has one-page care sheets on many other species
www.reptilesmagazine.com	Many care sheets, especially on less common species
www.kingsnake.com	Has information on many species, care sheets, and forums
www.iherp.com	Forums for owners to ask questions, also allows people to set up profiles and keep tracking information for their animals
www.greenigsociety.org www.iguanaden.org	Care information for green iguanas
www.beardeddragon.org	Care information for bearded dragons
www.triciaswaterdragon.com	Care information for Chinese water dragons
www.pangea.com	Care information for crested geckos and *Rhacodactylus* spp
www.tortoisetrust.org	Care information for box turtles and tortoises
www.russiantortoise.net	Care information mainly for Russian tortoises but has information that applies to many tortoise species
www.chameleoncare.net	Basic care information for chameleons

This list is not complete. These sources are sources the author has found useful for clients.

temperature extremes, or change of season; this may persist in captive specimens if not properly acclimated.[7]

Reptiles can generally be divided into 3 categories: carnivores, omnivores, and herbivores. Carnivores include all snakes and crocodilians, most monitors and tegus, the venomous lizards (*Heloderma* spp), and many other lizards, including the common pets leopard geckos (*Eublepharis macularius*) and most chameleons (some species will consume occasional plant matter). Omnivores include most turtles and lizards, such as box turtles, aquatic turtles, bearded dragons (*Pogona vitticeps*), Chinese water dragons (*Physignathus cocincinus*), and blue-tongued skinks (*Tiliqua* spp). Many omnivores change food preferences throughout their lives, being more carnivorous when young and incorporating more plant material into their diet as they age.[5,6] Herbivores include tortoises, green iguanas (*Iguana iguana*), and other iguana species (*Ctenosaurus* spp, *Cyclura* spp), *Uromastyx* spp, chuckwallas (*Sauromalus* spp), and prehensile-tailed skinks (*Corucia zebrata*). Herbivores rely on hindgut fermentation, similar to herbivorous mammals.[5,6]

Snakes are carnivores requiring a diet of whole prey. Depending on the species, this can be a variety of rodents, chicks, fish, frogs, toads, lizards, or even eggs, worms, and insects. The easiest prey item to obtain is rodents, and most snakes readily accept these. For picky snakes, such as young ball pythons (*Python regius*), sometimes alternative prey items will be accepted, such as a gerbil or African soft-furred mouse (*Mastomys natalensis*). There are some species that naturally feed on different prey animals, such as the hognose snakes (*Heterodon* spp) on toads, many kingsnake species (*Lampropeltis* spp) on lizards, and other kingsnakes and the king cobra (*Ophiophagus hannah*) on other snakes. These animals can often be converted to rodents by scent transfer of their preferred prey item onto a rodent. Rodents should preferably be fed frozen-thawed rather than live to prevent injury to the snake or possible parasite transmission. Presenting food on tongs is recommended to encourage the snake to engage in natural striking and coiling behavior. Snakes that are fed in their enclosures, especially from hands rather than tongs, often learn to exhibit a feeding response each time the enclosure is opened; feeding the snake in a separate enclosure can help prevent this.[6,8] Old laboratory rodents that have had multiple litters should not be fed as prey items, as they are often obese, resulting in an increased fat content for the snake.[6,7] Most snakes are typically fed once weekly to once monthly, depending on their size and life stage, though young, fast-moving snakes like garter snakes (*Thamnophis* spp) and mambas (*Dendroaspis* spp) need to be fed more often.[8]

Crocodilians are also carnivorous. A hatchling crocodilian's diet is primarily insects and a variety of small fish.[9] As they grow, their prey size increases and can include larger fish, birds, other reptiles, and mammals. Typically crocodilians in captivity should be fed once to twice weekly, whereas those in production farms are often fed daily to every other day.[9] A typical diet is beef, horse meat, fish, and/or poultry. Gharials are mainly fish eaters.[9,10] There are also some commercial diets available that are of good quality and produced in various sizes.[9,10]

Carnivorous lizards eat a variety of prey items. Monitors and tegus will readily accept rodents, chicks, and eggs; but care must be taken not to overfeed, as these species are extremely prone to obesity in captivity. A variety of insect prey items should be fed to monitors and tegus in addition to rodents and birds. Most other carnivorous lizards, such as geckos and chameleons, are insectivorous. A variety of insect prey items are available, such as crickets, mealworms, superworms, silk worms, phoenix worms, wax worms, roaches, moths, and fruit flies. The nutritional content of some of these prey items can be seen in **Table 2**. A variety of prey items should be offered

Table 2
Nutritional content of select invertebrate prey items

Insect	Protein (% DM)	Fat (% DM)	ME (kcal/kg)	Calcium (% DM)	Phosphorus (% DM)	Vitamin D₃ (IU/kg)	Vitamin A (IU/kg)
House cricket (Acheta domestica)	40–68	19–44	1402	0.1–0.2	0.8–1.4	<256	<1000
Mealworm (Tenebrio molitor)	35–55	31–60	1378	0.04–0.12	0.9–1.4	<256	<1000
Superworm (Zoophobas morio)	40–50	41–44	2423	0.03–0.12	0.6–0.8	<256	<1000
Waxworm (Galleria mellonella)	27–41	51–73	2747	0.06–0.07	0.6–1.2	<256	<1000
Silkworm (Bombyx mori)	65	4–21	674	0.21	0.54	<256	1580
Earthworm (Lumbricus terresstris)	73	11–13	708	1.2	0.86	<256	<1000
Fruit fly (Drosophila melanogaster)	68	19	—	0.17	1.32	—	2.2
Turkestan roach (Blatta lateralis)	76.05	14.45	—	0.24	1.22	—	120
Hissing cockroach (Gromphadorhina portentosa)	63.35	20.3	—	0.25	0.93	—	182
Wood lice (Porcellio scaber)	41.2	11.5	—	14.38	1.22	—	—

Abbreviations: DM, dry matter; ME, metabolizable energy.
Data from Refs.[6,50,51]

to provide the most well-balanced diet; unfortunately, most owners choose one or 2 insects to feed. Insects need to be fed complete diets and be supplemented in order to provide the best nutrition to the reptile. Insects should typically be fed to the reptile out of a dish or in a separate container to avoid accidental ingestion of bedding material. They should be no longer that the width of the reptile's head, and the reptile should only be fed what it can eat in one sitting, as many insects will bite the reptile if left in the enclosure. Some sources for feeders are listed in **Table 3**.

Herbivorous animals include many lizards and tortoises. Herbivorous lizards should be eating a mixture of dark leafy greens, such as collard greens, mustard greens, turnip greens, dandelion greens, escarole, endive, and watercress. Other greens can be fed occasionally to add variety to the diet. Some plants, such as kale, cabbage, or other cruciferous plants, are high in goitrogens, which bind iodine and can lead to goiter or hypothyroidism.[5–7,11] Others, such as spinach, rhubarb, beet greens, and cabbage, are high in oxalates, which bind calcium and inhibit its absorption.[5–7] Besides greens, a wide variety of shredded or chopped vegetables should also be offered. These vegetables can be items such as beans, peas, squashes, sweet potato, carrot, bell peppers, and zucchini. Fruit should be offered only occasionally, more as a treat. Most herbivores enjoy edible flowers as a treat as well, such as hibiscus, roses, or dandelions. Tortoises housed outdoors should primarily be grazing on vegetation and grasses; when kept indoors, grass hays can be offered in addition to the salad items described for lizards. Some tortoise species, such as the red-footed tortoise (Chelonoidis carbonaria), will naturally eat a small amount of animal protein as well,

Table 3 Sources of commonly used reptile products	
General reptile supply Web sites	www.lllreptile.com www.beanfarm.com www.reptiledirect.com www.bigappleherp.com
Manufacturers of reptile products, large variety of options	www.zoomed.com www.exo-terra.com
Enclosures	www.visionproducts.us www.npicages.com www.boaphileplastics.com www.glasscages.com www.waterlandtubs.com
Misting systems	www.mistking.com www.pro-products.com
Thermostats and supplies	www.spyderrobotics.com www.helixcontrols.com
Infrared noncontact temperature guns	www.tempgun.com www.raytek.com
UVB meters	www.solarmeter.com
Insect feeders	www.armstrongcrickets.com www.feedersource.com www.mulberryfarms.com
Rodent feeders	www.rodentpro.com www.americanrodent.com www.micedirect.com
Tortoise grass mixes, other foods, and insect feeders	www.carolinapetsupply.com

Adapted from Barten SL, Fleming GJ. Current herpetologic husbandry and products. In: Mader DR, Divers SJ, editors. Current therapy in reptile medicine and surgery. St Louis (MO): Elsevier Saunders; 2014. p. 2–12.

such as a pinkie mouse or insects; but this should be offered only once a month. Commercial diets are available for many herbivore species. Tortoise pellets made by Mazuri (Land O'Lakes, Inc, St Paul, MN) are nutritionally sound but should be offered no more than once a week as they contain higher protein and starch levels than typical grass browse.[12] Many commercial diets for herbivores and omnivores are not nutritionally complete, and any formula should be examined closely before feeding. Any dry pellets should be soaked in water before feeding and should only be used to supplement the diet not as a primary food source.

Omnivorous animals will typically eat a mixture of what has been described for carnivores and herbivores. Omnivorous lizards and box turtles should be offered a variety of insects and worms, besides the salad items listed. Lizards will also often accept pinkie mice as a treat. Aquatic turtles will eat a variety of insects, worms, and fish, along with shredded greens and vegetables. Aquatic turtle pellets are one of the few commercial diets that seem to be nutritionally complete, and these should make up most of the diet.[5,12,13] Live fish, such as minnows or goldfish, can also be fed as a supplement. When feeding aquatic turtles, it is important not to overfeed so that the water does not become soiled; feeding in a separate container can help avoid this.[13,14] Geckos native to New Caledonia (*Rhacodactylus* spp, *Correlophus ciliatus*) are becoming very popular as pets and have more unique nutritional requirements. In the wild, these geckos typically eat fruit that has fallen from trees and partially rotted on the ground, along with some insect material. This diet is obviously difficult to replicate in captivity, but several companies (Repashy Superfoods [San Marcos, CA]; Pangea Reptile [Grand Rapids, MI]) have developed diets made to mimic this natural diet. These diets should be made fresh every other day, with insects offered once a week to these lizards.

NUTRACEUTICALS

Most reptile diets, other than whole vertebrate prey, need some type of supplementation. Most supplements are typically provided in the form of powders that can be sprinkled or dusted onto food. Insects can be dusted with supplements that stick to the exoskeleton. However, they must be eaten immediately, as dust falls off or is groomed off by some insects, such as crickets.[5,6] Some lizard species will lick powdered calcium out of a dish, especially if the prey items are offered in the dish as well. Supplements can also be dusted on salad items, but some animals find these unpalatable, so they must be mixed in or the salad misted with water first to dissolve the powder. Gut loading is a process that involves feeding a high-calcium diet to invertebrate prey. However, it has been determined that this process may not significantly alter the nutritional content of the prey item or that it may increase the calcium content of the insect but cause fatal constipation before the insect can be consumed.[6,7,15] Instead, providing a high-quality diet to the insects is typically recommended along with proper supplementation.

Calcium is the mineral most often supplemented in reptile diets. Calcium is inadequate especially in invertebrate prey items (**Table 2**), and most need to be supplemented before feeding. Newborn mice are deficient in calcium as well; if this will be a long-term food source, calcium supplementation is recommended. Some sources state that allowing the mice to obtain milk from their mother for a day or two increases the calcium content, but this has not been proven.[5] Multiple types of calcium supplements may be provided, with calcium carbonate being the most readily available. Calcium included in multivitamin powders is typically not sufficient to meet the requirements.[5,6] Owners should also be wary of supplements that contain phosphorus and vitamin D_3. Supplements containing phosphorus typically negate the beneficial effects of calcium. Animals that spend time outdoors or under artificial UVB lighting do not need oral vitamin D_3 supplementation, and providing additional vitamin D_3 can lead to toxicity.[5,11] Nocturnal species that do not have access to UVB (such as many gecko species) should have vitamin D_3 included in their supplementation. Carnivorous reptiles obtain the vitamin D_3 they need through their diet of whole prey. Although the exact rate of calcium supplementation depends on the species and the diet provided, as a general rule it can be supplemented 3 to 5 times a week and then less often once the animal reaches its adult size. Less supplementation is needed if an animal is eating primarily a commercial diet.

Multivitamin supplements are essential to diets made of invertebrates and mixed salads as well. Many reptile owners are aware of the necessity of calcium supplementation but fail to provide other vitamins and minerals. There are many reptile products available, but some keepers and veterinarians advocate grinding and using human multivitamins instead as there is superior regulation on these products.[5] For most species, these supplements can be provided once a week.

Hypovitaminosis A has long been recognized as a problem in chelonians but only more recently in insectivorous lizards. Some animals possess enzymes that are capable of converting carotenoid precursors into retinol or retinal, both of which have vitamin A activity. Animals that do not possess these enzymes required preformed vitamin A in their diet. Preformed vitamin A is available in whole vertebrate prey, whereas carotenoid compounds are available in greens and vegetables. Herbivorous reptiles are able to convert these carotenoids in plant material to vitamin A. Although some insectivorous lizards are able to convert carotenoids to vitamin A, some are not, meaning that supplements containing preformed vitamin A must be used for these species.[16,17]

Vitamin B_1 (thiamine) and vitamin E supplementation is important for those species eating fish. Many fish species contain thiaminase, which breaks down thiamine in the fish.[5–7,11] Thiamine supplementation is especially important if frozen fish are being fed; thiamine must be supplemented. Fish also contain high levels of polyunsaturated fatty acids; steatitis from vitamin E deficiency is a possible outcome if this vitamin is not supplemented.[5–7,11]

HOUSING

Traditionally, stark, easily cleaned cages with nonparticulate substrate, a water bowl, and a hide box were recommended for most reptiles (**Fig. 1**A). The advantage of these types of enclosures is their ease of maintenance but at the cost of stimulation and enrichment.[1,8,18–21] Larger, more naturalistic enclosures are more commonly recommended now as they provide much greater benefits to the reptiles themselves (see **Fig. 1**B). However, the owner must be dedicated about keeping the enclosure clean and dry, otherwise a simpler cage setup is usually best for the health of the animal.[18,19] Sources for enclosures and other cage accessories are listed in **Table 3**.

Reptiles caged in small, stark cages are often seen pacing. Those that constantly pace or wander are likely under higher levels of stress, resulting in immunosuppression and disease.[1,18] Pacing also often leads to rostral abrasions, which can in turn cause stomatitis and anorexia.[1,22] Reptiles kept in small enclosures may be more heavily parasitized than their wild counterparts because of constant exposure to parasite ova.[1] They may also exhibit behaviors not typically seen in their wild counterparts.[1,22] Ideally, a reptile should find certain areas in its enclosure and stay there for periods of time. Numerous hiding, resting, and activity areas should be provided. Activities can include stimulating behaviors, such as foraging for food or water, seeking mates, thermoregulating, or seeking shelter.[1,23] In large outdoor enclosures, many reptiles will establish territories and defend them, even against their keepers, behaving more like wild reptiles.[1]

The enclosure for most reptiles should be as large as the owner can provide. Larger cages are associated with fewer self-inflicted injuries, better body condition, and

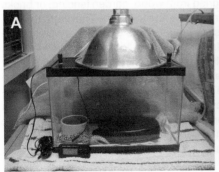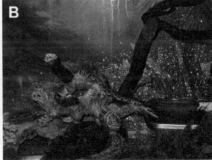

Fig. 1. (*A*) Typical sparsely furnished enclosure housing a leopard gecko (*Eublepharis macularius*). (*B*) Naturalistic enclosure for a ball python (*Python regius*). (*Courtesy of* Dan Johnson, DVM, DABVP (Exotic Companion Mammal), Raleigh, NC.)

higher rates of reproduction.[1,20,22] In general, enclosures with solid sides and tops are preferred as it is easier to maintain proper temperature and humidity levels. Materials that work well for this purpose are glass, plastic, plexiglass, stainless steel, and synthetic materials, such as fiberglass, melamine, or compressed polyvinyl chloride (PVC). These smooth materials are easier to disinfect and not as likely to cause rostral abrasions or other injuries.[1,18] Plywood is commonly used, but the rough surface is more likely to cause injury and is very difficult to disinfect or eliminate mites from.[1] If plywood is going to be used, it needs to be sealed with polyurethane or other water-proofing agents and then allowed to dry before putting a reptile inside it.[19] Glass aquariums are commonly used because they are easily available, but it is difficult to maintain proper heat and humidity for some species when using these enclosures as moisture and heat will rise out of the top.[20] Some reptiles, particularly Chinese water dragons (*Physignathus cocincinus*), also have difficulty with the clear glass and constantly rub their nose on the glass trying to escape.[1,22] Plastic storage tubs are often used for snakes or terrestrial turtles and tortoises, and these can work well as long as they are properly secured and of appropriate size. Many keepers with large collections of snakes use rack systems that consist of plastic storage tubs stacked on top of one another separated by shelves with heat tape in between. Although these cages are functional and easy to clean, they provide very little in terms of enrichment or exercise.[8,20] One notable exception to these rules are chameleons, who thrive in screen or wire mesh cages providing plenty of ventilation.

Terrestrial animals should have enclosures with a much larger floor space, and the enclosure needs sufficient height to allow the animal room to move around without coming in contact with overhead heat or light sources or escaping from the top.[1] Arboreal species should have a taller cage to allow plenty of space for climbing, but the size of the floor space is not as important. For lizards, the minimum cage recommendations are twice as long and one time as wide as the lizard is long and for arboreal species at least twice as high as the lizard is long.[19–21] One recommendation for snakes is that the enclosure length plus width is at least equal to the length of the snake.[20,21] Others suggest that a snake should be able to adopt a straight-line posture.[22] For chelonians, the shell should not exceed 25% of the floor space of the enclosure.[13] Large lizards and chelonians are often allowed to roam free in the house. Although many owners set up UVB and heat lamps for these animals to bask under, it is nearly impossible to maintain proper temperature and humidity with these free-roaming setups.

Many species do much better if kept outdoors; for some large species, such as crocodilians or giant tortoises, keeping them indoors is not an option. Small turtles and tortoises can do well in enclosures designed from wood, garden fencing, or bricks (**Fig. 2**A). There must be some type of wire mesh over the top of the enclosure to deter predators but still allow access to natural sunlight. Fire ants can also attack and kill tortoises kept outdoors.[14,24] Outdoor ponds are preferable for aquatic turtles. Large tortoises need fencing that is buried into the ground or they are able to dig under the fence or knock it over and escape. Terrestrial turtles and tortoises need some type of shelter (see **Fig. 2**B). In areas of the country with cold nights or winters, insulated doghouses or sheds that are heated should be provided.[14,21] Crocodilians almost invariably need to be kept in outdoor enclosures because of their size, though young animals may be kept indoors while they are growing. Typically, sturdy buried fencing is used with a large pond for swimming and a large land area used as a haul-out for basking.

Many reptile species require aquatic areas provided in the enclosure or even most of the enclosure devoted to water with a small land area. These areas can be created by adding large plastic tubs that can be easily removed for cleaning or by creating an area

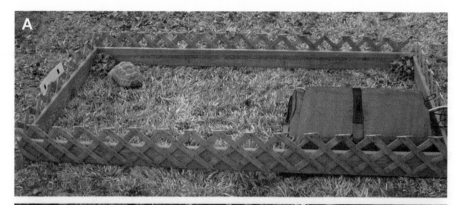

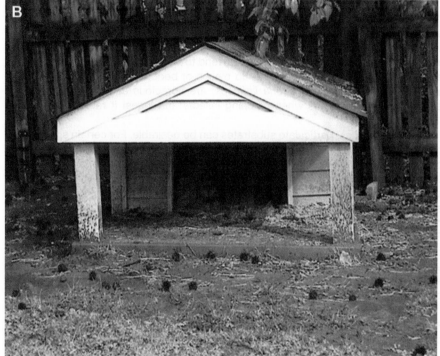

Fig. 2. (A) Outdoor enclosure set up with proper fencing and heated hide box appropriate for small tortoises. (B) Heated outdoor house for a Sulcata tortoise (*Geochelone sulcata*) within a fenced yard. (*Courtesy of* Dan Johnson, DVM, DABVP (Exotic Companion Mammal), Raleigh, NC.)

that can be drained and refilled, as many reptiles will soil their water frequently with fecal material or bedding. For species that are mostly aquatic, a dry land area should be provided that the animal can easily access for basking and drying off. The water should have excellent filtration, and regular water changes should be performed. As with keeping fish, there are beneficial bacteria in the water column that metabolize waste and help maintain water quality. These bacteria can be beneficial in keeping pathogenic bacteria in check and promoting good skin health.[1] For aquatic species, such as turtles and crocodilians, moving in and out of the water is a method of thermoregulation and osmoregulation as well.[9,13]

Almost all species benefit from some area of privacy. For most species, a hide box made from cardboard, pottery, PVC or plastic tubes, or bark works well to provide the animal a space to retreat. Most animals prefer smaller hide boxes in which they can touch most, if not all, of the sides.[25] For arboreal species, either real or artificial plants and leaves can be used to provide areas to hide up in the climbing branches in the enclosure. If the animal is not using the hide box, then something different should be tried. Some shy species will not eat and become stressed if they lack a secure place to hide.[18,19]

SUBSTRATE

The substrate used also varies based on the species, size of the animal, and usefulness of the material. Nonparticulate substrates, such as newspaper, paper towels, or carpet, are very easy to keep clean and are less expensive but are unattractive in a naturalistic enclosure. They also may not be appropriate for certain species, such as those who like to burrow. These types of substrates work well for young lizards who seem especially prone to ingesting particulate substrates and developing impactions. Green iguanas (*Iguana iguana*) tend to flick their tongues repeatedly while exploring their environment, picking up pieces of bedding material while doing so. Young bearded dragons (*Pogona vitticeps*) are voracious eaters that tend to get substrate in their mouths when catching insects and ingest it rather than spitting it out.

For many species, particulate substrates can be desirable. For certain species with high humidity needs, substrates, such as cypress mulch or shredded coconut fiber, can be kept damp in one portion of the cage. However, proper ventilation must be used with these types of substrates; they must be cleaned frequently to prevent fungal and bacterial growth.[1,8,21] For species that like to dig or burrow, aspen shavings, shredded paper, or recycled paper bedding can work well. Particulate substrates may also pose an impaction risk, be dusty or irritating, and be difficult to clean. Some bedding materials, such as cedar shavings, contain aromatic compounds that can irritate the eyes or respiratory tract.[1,19] Those made of larger pieces, such as crushed walnut shell or corncob, are a much greater risk for causing impaction.[19–21] A popular bedding sold for reptiles is calcium sand. Although these products claim to be digestible and a good source of calcium, the author has seen many cases, and many other cases are reported, of impaction resulting from this product (**Fig. 3**).[19] If sand is desired for an enclosure, such as for animals that burrow like sand boas or other adult desert reptiles, then play sand is recommended because of the fine particle size. Again, the natural environment of the species needs to be taken into account. Substrates that are too acidic, too basic, too dry, too moist, or dirty contribute to dermatologic and respiratory problems in captive reptiles.[1,19,21] If using particulate substrates, one should also provide an area of tile, smooth rock, or carpet for offering food to help reduce the risk of accidental ingestion of the substrate.[20]

Bioactive substrates are becoming more widely used as well but have some distinct benefits and disadvantages. The theory behind these substrates is they provide an environment where beneficial bacteria compete with pathogenic bacteria and fungi to support a healthy microhabitat.[1,18,21,26] Stirring the substrate frequently is key, as it mixes the beneficial bacteria from the lower layers with the fecal bacteria on the upper layers, inhibiting their growth.[1,20,26] The substrate must be at least 6.5 cm (2.5 in) deep and allow for good oxygenation and moisture retention.[1,26] This type of substrate has been tested mainly on snakes also as a method to help control cutaneous water loss and prevent chronic dehydration when kept on dry substrates.[1,26]

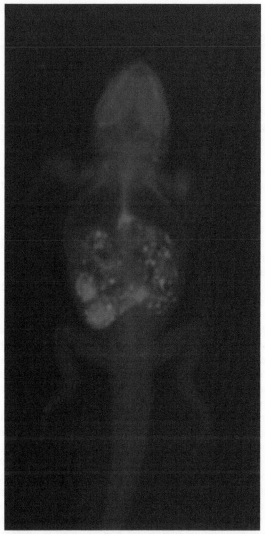

Fig. 3. Radiograph of a juvenile bearded dragon (*Pogona vitticeps*) with a gastrointestinal impaction from calcium sand bedding. (*Courtesy of* Dan Johnson, DVM, DABVP (Exotic Companion Mammal), Raleigh, NC.)

It would likely be useful for many other species as well; the author has seen it used successfully for small snakes, New Caledonian gecko species, and other arboreal species.

There are several generalizations that can be made when choosing a substrate. Turtles and tortoises tend to do well on loose substrates, such as cypress mulch, compressed straw pellets, or even rabbit pellets. Close attention must be paid to be sure the substrate is not staying too wet or becoming moldy. Aquatic turtles are notorious for eating small pea gravel if used in the bottom of their enclosure.[20] They typically do best with no substrate at all or by using stones larger than their head to prevent ingestion. Most snakes do well on newspaper, paper towels, aspen shavings, or cypress mulch, depending on size and species.[1,8] Most young lizards do best on newspaper,

paper towels, or carpet. Once they are older (depending on species), an area of sand or other particulate substrate can be provided in the enclosure as long as there is a clean area for feeding.

WATER AND HUMIDITY

Methods of water regulation vary among groups of reptiles, and once again research into an animal's native habitat must be done to determine the proper way to provide water and humidity in an enclosure. Generally speaking, animals from arid environments are uricotelic, producing large, insoluble molecules of uric acid in an attempt to conserve water.[1,3,5,7] Reptiles from aquatic environments produce smaller, more soluble urea, or even ammonia, to eliminate nitrogenous wastes.[1,3,5,7] Many use different combinations of these methods. All reptiles seem to engage in microhabitat selection, or choosing areas with varying levels of humidity, in order to combat insensitive water loss.[1,3] Reducing these water losses seems to be very important in combating long-term health problems, especially the development of renal disease.[1,3,7,25] Difficulty shedding also occurs if humidity is too low. In captive tortoises, higher levels of humidity are important in preventing growth deformities, such as pyramiding.[24,27]

Different species of reptiles drink water using various methods. Snakes will readily drink from a bowl, and the bowl should be large enough for them to soak in as well. Lizards and tortoises often have to learn how to drink from a water bowl, but when soaked in shallow water will drink readily.[1,7,11,14,24] Some species, such as crested geckos (*Correlophus ciliatus*) and anoles (*Anolis* spp), prefer to drink water droplets that collect on the sides of the enclosure during misting.[7,11,25] Chameleons drink best from a dripper system set up to collect droplets of water on leaves with a catch pan at the bottom of the cage.[11,21] There are commercial dripper systems available for this purpose, or they can be made from an intravenous fluid bag and drip set or a plastic bottle with a small hole in it.

Providing appropriate humidity can sometimes be a challenge, and providing appropriate humidity levels without encouraging bacterial and fungal growth can be difficult. By increasing ventilation to try to prevent this, often humidity levels can decrease, so a balance must be struck. In general, glass aquariums with screen tops are not appropriate reptile enclosures as they allow moisture and heat to escape out the top. Enclosures with solid sides are much better at maintaining humidity, with small areas on the sides added for ventilation. Axial fans, used to provide spot cooling for electronics, are now being incorporated into reptile enclosures as well.[20] Human humidifiers or vaporizers can be used in enclosures or by using PVC pipe to create a track that directs the mist into the enclosure. Commercial reptile foggers and misters are also sold for this purpose. These systems need to be cleaned regularly to avoid illness from bacterial growth.[20] Misting the tank can be done as well, but that is more effective for increasing humidity for a temporary time; to maintain a constant level of humidity, the tank would have to be misted many times per day.

Providing high humidity in select areas works well to meet the humidity needs of the reptiles. It allows them to move between microhabitats and helps prevent bacterial and fungal growth in the enclosure. A moist hide box can be created by using a plastic container with a lid on it, with a hole cut in the side or the lid for the animal to enter the box. Sphagnum moss, a washcloth, or paper towels inside the box should be kept damp to provide high humidity. This practice works especially well for certain reptiles like leopard geckos (*Eublepharis macularius*) or blue-tongued skinks (*Tiliqua* spp) to assist with ecdysis. Sometimes appropriate substrate, such as moss or mulch, can also be kept damp in a corner of the cage to provide increased humidity; this is commonly used for select snake species.

TEMPERATURE

Reptiles are ectothermic, meaning they rely on the temperature of their environment to regulate their own body temperature.[1,3,7] Most aspects of a reptile's physiology depend on temperature; the use of thermal gradients in the environment is especially important for a reptile's overall health. Most species have a preferred optimum temperature range (POTR) at which they thrive. The POTR for common veterinary patients are listed in **Table 4**. The immune response of reptiles varies on a seasonal basis and is intimately associated with environmental temperature.[1,4] Cellular and humoral immune responses are lower during winter months; therefore, reptiles may be more susceptible to disease during this time and if they are kept at temperatures too low for their species.[1]

A thermal gradient should be provided for every captive reptile, allowing the reptile to thermoregulate through natural behaviors. Temperatures should be higher during

Table 4
POTR for commonly kept species

Common Name	Scientific Name	Preferred Optimum Temperature Range (°F)
Boa constrictor	*Boa constrictor*	Mid 80s
Ball python	*Python regius*	Mid 80s
Burmese python	*Python molurus*	Mid 80s
Green tree python	*Morelia viridis*	75–82
Carpet python	*Morelia spilota*	80–85
Cornsnake	*Pantherophis guttatus*	77–84
Gopher or bullsnake	*Pituophis catenifer*	77–84
Kingsnakes	Lampropeltis spp	77–84
Green iguana	*Iguana iguana*	84–90
Leopard gecko	*Eublepharis macularius*	77–85
Day geckos	*Phelsuma* spp	85
Chameleons (montane)	*Chamaeleo* spp, *Trioceros jacksonii*	77–84
Chameleons (lowland)	*Chameleo* spp, *Furcifer pardalis*	80–84
Bearded dragons	*Pogona* spp	84–90
Blue-tongued skinks	*Tiliqua* spp	80–85
Monitors	*Varanus* spp	84–88
Crested gecko	*Correlophus ciliatus*	70–75
Aquatic turtles	Most species	80–84
Box turtles	*Terrapene* spp	78–89
Tortoises	Most species	82–88
Crocodilians	Most species	77–95

Note that this chart includes POTR only. Many species need a basking area that is warmer than these temperatures and a cooler side of the enclosure with lower temperatures.
From Rossi JV. General husbandry and management. In: Mader DR, editor. Reptile medicine and surgery. St Louis (MO): Saunders; 2006. p. 26, with permission.

the day and drop at night to provide natural variation. Seasonal variation should also be provided for animals that brumate. A variety of products are available to heat an enclosure. Under-tank heaters or radiant heat sources are most commonly used to provide a higher temperature in the POTR, but animals can move away from this to other areas in the enclosure to thermoregulate properly. The type of heat source used varies on the species being kept. Animals that bask, such as many lizards and chelonians, along with other arboreal reptiles, typically benefit from a radiant heat source from above, such as an incandescent light bulb, ceramic heat emitter, or heat panel. Aquatic species should have a submersible heater in the water but also a basking area. Under-tank heat sources can be appropriate for some species, such as snakes and many geckos, but they must be set up appropriately to avoid burns. The author commonly treats burns on the ventrum of snakes kept in glass aquariums with under-tank heaters as the snake will lie on the heat source trying to warm to its POTR, and burns develop before that temperature is reached.[22] Similar injuries occur with hot rocks, and these products should be avoided. Crocodilians typically regulate their body temperature by moving in and out of the water.[9] Decreasing the temperature at night is recommended to provide a more natural environment. For most species, nighttime temperatures should not decrease to less than 70°F (21°C). If nighttime heating is required, ceramic heat emitters work well for this purpose as they provide heat but no light.

The owner needs to monitor the temperature minimally on both sides of the enclosure but preferably throughout. Most stick-on thermometers sold by pet stores are not very accurate, and owners have a tendency to put them high up on the sides of the enclosure and not where the animal actually spends time. Digital thermometers with probes or infrared noncontact temperature guns are far more accurate and easier to use. Thermostats or rheostats can also be used to control temperature of an individual heat source in an enclosure.

Many temperate and montane species brumate (hibernate) at certain times of the year. This behavior is most common in snakes, temperate box and aquatic turtles, and some tortoises. This change is natural, and many keepers will observe their animals gradually starting to become less active and reducing their food intake. To prepare for brumation, an animal should be held off food, but maintained at its proper temperature, until its gastrointestinal tract is empty. The temperature can then gradually be lowered over several days to a week to the desired brumation temperature.[1,8] For most species, this is 40°F to 55°F (4.5°C–13°C) for approximately 3 months.[1,8,14] Snakes can typically be maintained in a plastic storage container on newspaper with water, but chelonians need to be provided with soil or mulch in which to bury themselves.[8,14] Chelonians can also brumate outdoors in an artificial burrow with plenty of loose substrate; if brumating outdoors, this period typically lasts 5 to 6 months.[14] For many species, especially temperate snakes, this temperature change is needed to stimulate breeding behaviors.[8,25] Tropical reptiles should not be brumated, though some (especially boas and pythons) require a decrease in nighttime temperatures for reproductive cycling.[1,8] Some temperate species of chelonians may skip brumation if temperatures and day length are kept the same all year round.[14] Brumation is only recommended for animals in good health and body weight.

LIGHTING

Photoperiod is important for reptiles for normal behavior and reproduction.[1,8,21,22] In general, the day length should correspond to natural lighting outdoors, providing longer days in the summer and decreasing the day length during the winter. Failure to change the day length and temperature can result in reproductive failure or disease in many reptiles.[1,3,21,25] Obesity can also be a sequela, as animals that would normally be inactive and not eat during the winter may continue eating if the photoperiod and temperature are not changed.[1] Electric timers can easily be used to provide a constant photoperiod. Providing access to natural lighting can also help to provide a more natural photoperiod, and animals typically respond more strongly to this than to artificial lighting.[1] Some keepers prefer to use a 12-hours-on/12-hours-off light cycle all year round; that can be suitable for some species, especially if there is no intention of breeding.

The quality of lighting is extremely important. Lighting in the UVA wavelength (320–400 nm) is generally provided, at least to some degree, by most light sources and can aid in stimulating natural behaviors.[1,21] UVB lighting (290–320 nm) is required for most captive reptiles. Exposure to UVB causes the cutaneous development of vitamin D_3, in turn allowing absorption of calcium from the intestinal tract. Without exposure to UVB lighting, nutritional secondary hyperparathyroidism is a common sequela. Basking reptiles benefit greatly from time outside in natural sunlight. Although exposure to natural sunlight is beneficial for reptiles, it must not be blocked by glass or plastic in order to be effective for vitamin D_3 production. Usually placing them in a small wire cage works best for this, as many tame reptiles will become agitated or aggressive and difficult to hold when exposed to natural sunlight.[19,21] No artificial bulb can fully replicate the sun, so animals that live in areas where they can be kept outdoors most of the year typically have better growth, health, behavior, reproduction, and longevity than those kept indoors.[19]

The exact UVB requirements for each species are largely unknown, though studies quantifying UVB exposure and vitamin D_3 levels are helpful in starting to determine the recommendations.[28–32] Basking species with high UVB requirements include bearded dragons, uromastyx, chuckwallas, green iguanas, and many tortoises.[20] There is a long held belief that snakes and nocturnal species do not need exposure to UVB when fed sufficient vitamin D_3 in the diet. Although these animals can be kept and bred successfully without UVB, anecdotal evidence suggests there are benefits seen, especially with reproduction.[20] Some recent studies show mixed results as to snakes and nocturnal species' ability to make vitamin D_3 with exposure to UVB lighting.[28–30] Panther chameleons (*Furcifer pardalis*) have been shown to adjust their exposure to UVB based on their vitamin D_3 levels, lending support to the theory that UVB gradients (just like temperature gradients) should potentially exist in an enclosure as well.[31,33]

There are 3 main types of UVB bulbs commercially available to reptile owners: fluorescent tubes, mercury vapor bulbs, and compact fluorescent bulbs. The type of bulb chosen depends on the species kept and the setup of the enclosure. Fluorescent tubes are available with different output levels of UVB, the higher levels being more suited for basking species and lower levels for nocturnal animals or those living mostly in shade. In general, these bulbs need to be placed closer than 12 in (30 cm) to the animal and may need to be replaced as often as every 6 to 8 months. They also do not produce heat. One can increase the output by providing 2 bulbs side by side in a fixture or by adding reflective material inside the fixture. There are newer tubes on the market, such as the ZooMed T5 HO UVB lamps (Zoo Med Laboratories, San Luis Obispo, CA), that can be placed further away and still be effective for vitamin D_3 production. Mercury vapor bulbs are usually recommended to be placed at least 12 in (30 cm) away from the reptile (sometimes further), and they provide heat, UVA, and UVB all in one bulb. Compact fluorescent bulbs produce UVB in only a very small area and do not produce heat. In general, this type of bulb is not very useful for a basking species because of its area of output. When these bulbs first became available, there was a high incidence of photokeratoconjunctivitis and photodermatitis associated with their use caused by a problem with the glass in the bulb allowing more short-wavelength UV radiation to penetrate.[34] Since this problem was discovered, it has largely been resolved, but the author still sees sporadic cases from time to time.

The Solarmeter UV Meter 6.2 and 6.5 (Solartech, Harrison Township, MI) are the most commonly used meters available to measure the UVB output of reptile lamps. The 6.2 m measures the amount of UVB in microwatts per square centimeter produced by the lamp, whereas the 6.5 m measures the UV index or the intensity. The combination of meters can help the clinician and owner determine the best areas of the cage to place basking perches and which types of bulb to use for their enclosure. These meters also allow a clinician to test a client's UVB bulb to know if it is still beneficial for the animal or needs to be replaced. In general, a bulb should be replaced when its output decrease to less than 70% of the initial readings for that lamp.[20]

ENVIRONMENTAL ENRICHMENT

Enrichment and training are widely accepted and implemented practices in zoos and aquaria but can also be incorporated into a reptile's care in private homes. Enrichment means encouraging species-appropriate behaviors and providing the animal with choices in every aspect of husbandry, thus enhancing animal welfare.[23] The goals for enrichment are to promote species-appropriate behaviors, provide behavioral opportunities, and to provide animals with control of their environment.[23,35,36] Other goals include reducing sources of chronic stress and reducing or eliminating aberrant behaviors.[35,36] Each of these goals requires a clear understanding of the animal's natural history in order to make the enrichment successful.

As discussed previously, providing large, more naturalistic enclosures for reptiles is now the standard recommended practice. Providing different levels, rocks, branches, plants, and substrates within the enclosure can encourage climbing, burrowing, and other more natural behaviors. These environmental changes also allow a reptile more choice in microhabitat selection, with exposure to different levels of light, heat, and humidity.[23] Elaborate setups can be constructed with products that are available now, with varying levels of heat, light, and humidity made available to the reptile that can stimulate certain times of day or even certain weather patterns.[25,37]

Historically reptiles have not been the focus on learning and enrichment as they were considered to not be as intelligent or capable of learning as other species, particularly mammals and birds. There is now evidence that shows that reptiles are not only capable of learning but some are also eager to participate in training schemes and complex behaviors can be shaped (see subsequent section on training).[38,39] There is also evidence that demonstrates that reptiles in enriched enclosures learn faster, habituate more quickly, and benefit greatly in other ways, such as becoming more active and exhibiting more natural behaviors.[38,40,41] Giving animals objects to play with is a common form of enrichment but is typically reserved for birds and mammals. Reptiles are stimulated by novel objects in the environment, but there is some evidence to suggest that they may be capable of play as well.[38,42]

FORAGING

One behavioral goal for enrichment may be to encourage foraging. Foraging provides one method of exercise along with mental stimulation. To encourage carnivores to forage, natural scents can be provided by dragging a prey item through the enclosure.[25,37] One can also bury that prey item, encouraging the reptile to dig to find it.[37] Sometimes novel scents can be used to stimulate a reptile, such as using cinnamon to encourage foraging in a Komodo dragon (*Varanus komodoensis*).[23] One can also vary the way the food is presented, such as varying the size, placement of the food, or time of day.[23] Live fish can be used for aquatic turtles and other partially aquatic species, such as garter snakes (*Thamnophis* spp) and Chinese water dragons (*Physignathus cocincinus*). Live insects should be provided for insectivores, as most of these animals hunt based on movement. One group found that foraging increased and aggression between conspecifics decreased when a slow-release cricket feeder was added to the enclosure.[43] Opened live fruit or insect-attracting lights could be placed in the enclosure to attract insects that a reptile may not normally have access to, though care must be taken to ensure this would not be harmful to the animal.[25] A variety of live plants can also be used for herbivores.[35,37] The author has successfully stimulated foraging in iguanas by using clips attached to the ceiling or sides of the enclosure to hold entire leaves of greens, mimicking tearing food from a tree or bush; this technique would work for other herbivores as well. Whole heads of greens, carrots, pumpkins, or squashes can be offered to tortoises; they will often spend more time eating from these than from their regular chopped salad mixture.[37] Offering live mammal or avian prey for carnivores can pose some inherent safety risks to the reptile or be deemed inhumane for the prey item. For these species, tease feeding a frozen thawed prey item on tongs can be used instead.[22,37] Providing different levels in an enclosure can also stimulate foraging. Monitors often stand bipedal to forage in the wild; this can be recreated by providing food items on different levels in an enclosure.[23]

WEIGHT MANAGEMENT

Reptiles in small enclosures do not have as much room to move around and often become heavier or overweight because of their reduced activity.[1,21] Enrichment can also provide ways for the reptile to exercise, thus helping the keeper control the animal's weight. One simple way to achieve this is to provide larger enclosures that give the animal more room for roaming and more levels and braches for climbing to exhibit natural behaviors. Climbing structures can also be available outside the enclosure (**Fig. 4**). The foraging techniques described earlier also encourage more activity and exercise. Chasing live food and following scent trails encourages exercise. Tease-feeding snakes by presenting frozen thawed prey items on tongs encourages the snake to strike and coil around the prey items, using muscles they may not if the prey item is just left in the enclosure. The environment should challenge the animal's body to maintain its physical strength.[35] In order to maintain proper body condition, consideration must be given to proper diet and feeding frequency as well.

BEHAVIOR TRAINING FOR HEALTHY INTERACTION WITH OWNERS

Training often goes hand in hand with enrichment. Operant conditioning can be used to train exotic animals, including reptiles, for husbandry purposes. This training helps facilitate daily care, capture and restraint, and medical procedures.[23,44] Many reptile species are naturally wary of humans and may react aggressively toward them. Training them to be accepting of handling may be necessary for them to receive proper care as a captive specimen, especially for pets in a private household. Many species can be trained to calmly enter a crate for a food reward in order to be transported rather than being physically restrained.[23,44,45] Monitor lizards, crocodilians, and tortoises have been conditioned to enter a crate; venomous snakes can be conditioned to enter a shift box.[23,44–46] Animals can also be trained to accept some medical

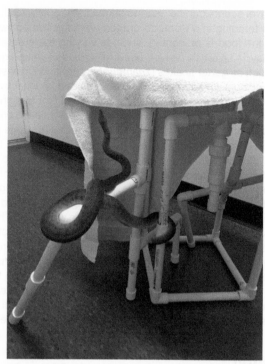

Fig. 4. Children's python (*Antaresia childreni*) using a climbing structure for exercise and enrichment outside of its enclosure. (*Courtesy of* Leigh Clayton, DVM, DABVP (Avian, Reptile and Amphibian), Baltimore, MD.)

procedures, such as ultrasounds, venipuncture, injections, and nail clipping.[23,44,47] Target training can also be used with reptiles; once they are trained to target, additional behaviors can be shaped as well (**Fig. 5**).[44,47,48]

To create a training plan, many facilities use the SPIDER (setting goals, planning, implementing, documenting, evaluating, and readjusting) framework taught by the Association of Zoos and Aquaria.[23,36] During goal setting, one must detail the specific behavior to be trained and how it benefits the keeper, the reptile, and potentially the veterinarian. The planning stage is when the series of steps for shaping the behavior is determined, and then these steps are implemented in the next stage. The keeper will then document how training sessions are progressing by keeping written notes or recording the sessions on video. The last 2 steps require evaluation of the documentation and making any changes necessary to achieve the behavioral goals.

Desensitization is also used in training reptiles. Desensitization is the process of getting an animal used to a new stimulus through gradual exposure to it.[44] This process can be done passively, such as by putting something new in an enclosure, or actively with involvement from a trainer.[44] The most common example of desensitization is handling. Over time animals can become accustomed to being touched in a certain way, then being picked up, then be conditioned to allow other types of handling or procedures.[44] They should receive a cue that handling is about to occur and never be surprised so as not to damage the trust between animal and handler.[44] Snakes who are fed in their enclosure often learn to associate a hand entering their enclosure for any reason with food and may strike. This behavior is unacceptable to the owner who wants to handle their snake. Although feeding snakes in a separate enclosure

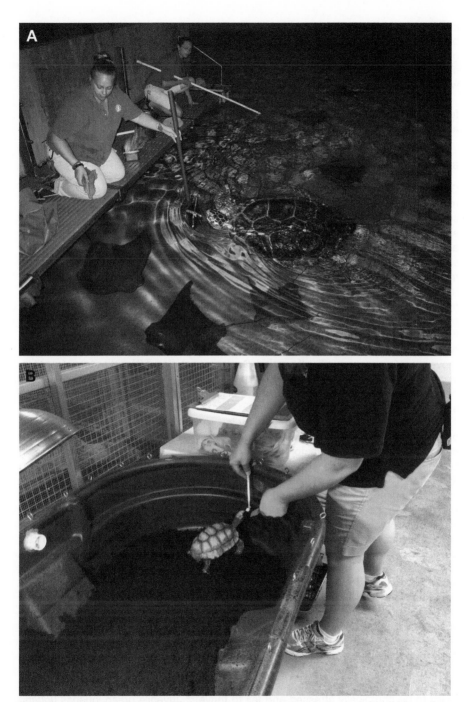

Fig. 5. Target training being used in (*A*) a green sea turtle (*Chelonia mydas*) and (*B*) a yellow-footed tortoise (*Chelonoidis denticulata*). (*Courtesy of* Leigh Clayton, DVM, DABVP (Avian, Reptile and Amphibian), Baltimore, MD.)

can help to alleviate this behavior, another option is to give the snake a cue that it is not being fed. Taking the snake out of the enclosure using a snake hook is one option, as is gently placing a towel over the snake's head when entering the enclosure. By desensitizing the snake to the new stimulus, either of these objects can then be removed with the snake remaining calm for handling rather than striking for food.

More detailed information on setting up enrichment and training programs can be found on Disney Animal Program's enrichment and training Web sites at www. animalenrichment.org and www.animaltraining.org, respectively.

BEHAVIOR TRAINING FOR HEALTHY INTERACTION WITH CONSPECIFICS

Group housing or multi-pet households with interaction between conspecifics is common in social animals, such as mammals and birds; however, many reptiles are solitary in the wild. Although social interaction can be a form of enrichment for social species, group housing can often create undo stress in reptiles. Training reptiles to accept conspecifics may not be a feasible goal for some species. In hatchling snapping turtles (Chelydra serpentina) and juvenile American alligators (Alligator mississippiensis), growth was slower and corticosterone levels were higher when raised with high stocking densities.[25,49] In the wild, reptiles would certainly encounter members of their own species and other species. These diverse auditory, gustatory, olfactory, visual, and other stimuli certainly affect their response to their environment, whether negatively or positively.[25] These factors should be considered when designing enclosures, as animals must be given enough space and retreats to move away from conspecifics if needed. Sometimes mixing different orders of reptiles, such as arboreal lizards with terrestrial or aquatic chelonians, can be done with proper planning and awareness of behaviors and disease; in some cases, this may be quite stimulating for the animals involved.[37]

Social behavior among snakes typically involves reproductive activity. During this time, a snake's behavior can change considerably; courtship, mating, and combat can all be observed.[8] Olfactory stimuli seem especially important to snakes in breeding, so removing the female and replacing her in the male's enclosure or leaving the female's shed skins in the enclosure can provide mental stimulation for the male.[25] In zoos multispecies exhibits are common, and they typically house multiple species that occupy different niches of the same ecosystem (terrestrial, arboreal, aquatic, and so forth) to avoid competition for resources. One must be careful during feeding time when housing multiple snakes in one enclosure as injuries or even cannibalism can occur. If both snakes attempt to swallow the same prey item, one may keep going and ingest the other snake, killing both of them.[8] Ophiophagus species, such as kingsnakes (Lampropeltis spp), must be watched very closely when introduced for breeding as one will often attempt to eat the other.[8]

In general, most lizards are highly territorial and are stressed by the presence of conspecifics, though some lizards have highly complex social structures.[19,22,38] Males are more territorial than females and react more violently to the presence of another male; this is especially true during breeding season.[19] When 2 lizards are kept together, one may physically attack the other inflicting serious injuries. Often one may dominate the other by keeping it away from the food and heat sources, causing the subordinate lizard to be chronically stressed and fail to thrive.[19] Juvenile green iguanas (Iguana iguana) have been shown to avoid the femoral secretions of adult conspecifics, a factor that should be considered when housing animals of different ages.[25] Adding additional food sources at unpredictable times can help increase activity and decrease aggression between animals.[43]

Certain species of chelonians may be aggressive to other turtles and conspecifics, such as snapping turtles, large softshell turtles, and bigheaded turtles.[14] Some male tortoises can be aggressive to other males, even fighting and trying to flip one another.[14]

In the wild, crocodilians are typically solitary predators, coming together for breeding. However, in captivity, small groups are commonly maintained in large enclosures without incident. Behaviors such as vocalization, aggressiveness, movement, dominance/submissiveness, and thermoregulation are all observed.[9] Hatchlings and young crocodilians tend to form social groups, more for safety, and do not exhibit any form of dominance.[9] Adults, however, form a definite social order within the group, which depends on vocalizations, postures, odors, and physical contact.[9] Crocodilians also exhibit parental care, which is fairly uncommon among reptiles. Crocodilians also use more vocalizations than most other reptile species, so providing recordings of conspecifics or young could provide enrichment as well.[25,37]

Captive reptile care has made many advances in recent years. Proper husbandry is the most important factor in keeping reptiles healthy. Providing proper nutrition, caging, lighting, temperature, substrate, and humidity are necessary otherwise disease can result. Providing larger, more naturalistic enclosures is recommended for reptiles to provide enrichment and more exhibition of natural behaviors. Through enrichment and training, one can improve the captive welfare of their animal along with their relationship with that animal.

REFERENCES

1. Rossi JV. General husbandry and management. In: Mader DR, editor. Reptile medicine and surgery. St Louis (MO): Saunders; 2006. p. 25–41.
2. Denardo D. Stress in captive reptiles. In: Mader DR, editor. Reptile medicine and surgery. St Louis (MO): Saunders; 2006. p. 119–23.
3. Lillywhite HB, Gatten RE. Physiology and functional anatomy. In: Warwick C, Frye FL, Murphy JB, editors. Health and welfare of captive reptiles. London: Chapman and Hall; 1995. p. 6–31.
4. Guillette LJ, Cree A, Rooney AA. Biology of stress: interactions with reproduction, immunology, and intermediary metabolism. In: Warwick C, Frye FL, Murphy JB, editors. Health and welfare of captive reptiles. London: Chapman and Hall; 1995. p. 32–81.
5. Stahl S, Donoghue S. Nutrition of reptiles. In: Hand MS, Thatcher CD, Remillard RL, et al, editors. Small animal clinical nutrition. Topeka (KS): Mark Morris Institute; 2010. p. 1237–49.
6. Donoghue S. Nutrition. In: Mader DR, editor. Reptile medicine and surgery. St Louis (MO): Saunders; 2006. p. 251–98.
7. Donoghue S, McKeown S. Nutrition of captive reptiles. Vet Clin North Am Exot Anim Pract 1999;2:69–91.
8. Funk RS. Snakes. In: Mader DR, editor. Reptile medicine and surgery. St Louis (MO): Saunders; 2006. p. 42–58.
9. Lane T. Crocodilians. In: Mader DR, editor. Reptile medicine and surgery. St Louis (MO): Saunders; 2006. p. 100–17.
10. Fleming GJ. Crocodiles and allies – what a practitioner should know. Proceedings of the North American Veterinary Conference. Orlando (FL): 2007. p. 1531–5.
11. Frye FL. Nutritional considerations. In: Warwick C, Frye FL, Murphy JB, editors. Health and welfare of captive reptiles. London: Chapman and Hall; 1995. p. 82–97.

12. Fleming GJ. Reptile nutrition – what's new?. Proceedings of the North American Veterinary Conference. Orlando (FL): 2007. p. 1536–7.
13. Johnson JH. Husbandry and medicine of aquatic reptiles. Semin Avian Exot Pet Med 2004;13:223–8.
14. Boyer TH, Boyer DM. Turtles, tortoises, and terrapins. In: Mader DR, editor. Reptile medicine and surgery. St Louis (MO): Saunders; 2006. p. 78–99.
15. Finke MD. Gut loading to enhance the nutrient content of insects as food for reptiles: a mathematical approach. Zoo Biol 2003;22:147–62.
16. Boyer TH, Garner MM, Reavill DR, et al. Common problems of leopard geckos (Eublepharis macularius). Proceedings of the Association of Reptilian and Amphibian Veterinarians conference. Indianapolis (IN): 2013. p. 17–25.
17. Dierenfeld ES, Norkus EB, Carroll K, et al. Carotenoids, vitamin A, and vitamin E concentrations during egg development in panther chameleons (Furcifer pardalis). Zoo Biol 2002;21:295–303.
18. Warwick C, Steedman C. Naturalistic versus clinical environments in husbandry and research. In: Warwick C, Frye FL, Murphy JB, editors. Health and welfare of captive reptiles. London: Chapman and Hall; 1995. p. 113–30.
19. Barten SL. Lizards. In: Mader DR, editor. Reptile medicine and surgery. St Louis (MO): Saunders; 2006. p. 59–77.
20. Barten SL, Fleming GJ. Current herpetologic husbandry and products. In: Mader DR, Divers SJ, editors. Current therapy in reptile medicine and surgery. St Louis (MO): Elsevier Saunders; 2014. p. 2–12.
21. De Vosjoli P. Designing environments for captive amphibians and reptiles. Vet Clin North Am Exot Anim Pract 1999;2:43–68.
22. Warwick C. Psychological and behavioral principles and problems. In: Warwick C, Frye FL, Murphy JB, editors. Health and welfare of captive reptiles. London: Chapman and Hall; 1995. p. 205–38.
23. Fleming GJ, Skurski ML. Conditioning and behavioral training in reptiles. In: Mader DR, Divers SJ, editors. Current therapy in reptile medicine and surgery. St Louis (MO): Elsevier Saunders; 2014. p. 128–32.
24. Innis CJ. Chelonian species identification and husbandry recommendations. Exotic DVM 2004;6:57–63.
25. Hayes MP, Jennings MR, Mellen JD. Beyond mammals: environmental enrichment for amphibians and reptiles. In: Shepherson DJ, Mellen JD, Hutchins M, editors. Second nature: environmental enrichment for captive animals. Washington, DC: Smithsonian Institution; 1998. p. 205–35.
26. De Vosjoli P. The art of keeping snakes. Irvine (CA): Advanced Vivarium Systems; 2004.
27. Wiesner CS, Iben C. Influence of environmental humidity and dietary protein on pyramidal growth of carapaces in African spurred tortoises (Geochelone sulcata). J Anim Physiol Anim Nutr 2003;87:66–74.
28. Acierno MJ, Mitchell MA, Zachariah TT, et al. Effects of ultraviolet radiation on plasma 25-hydroxyvitamin D3 concentrations in corn snakes (Elaphe [Pantherophis] guttata). Am J Vet Res 2008;69:294–7.
29. Hedley J, Eatwell K. Effects of UVB radiation on plasma 25-hydroxy vitamin D3 and ionized calcium concentrations in ball pythons (Python regius). Proceedings of the Association of Reptilian and Amphibian Veterinarians conference. Indianapolis (IN): 2013. p. 108.
30. Wangen K, Kirchenbaum J, Mitchell MA. Measuring 25-hydroxy vitamin D levels in leopard geckos exposed to commercial ultraviolet B lights. Proceedings of the

Association of Reptilian and Amphibian Veterinarians conference. Indianapolis (IN): 2013. p. 42.

31. Ferguson GW, Brinker AM, Karsten KB, et al. Voluntary exposure of some western-hemisphere snake and lizard species to ultraviolet-B radiation in the field: how much ultraviolet-B should a lizard or snake receive in captivity? Zoo Biol 2010;29:317–34.

32. Acierno MJ, Mitchell MA, Roundtree MK, et al. Effects of ultraviolet radiation on plasma 25-hydroxyvitamin D3 synthesis in red-eared slider turtles (Trachemys scripta elegans). Am J Vet Res 2006;67:2046–9.

33. Ferguson GW, Gehrmann WH, Karsten KB, et al. Do panther chameleons bask to regulate endogenous vitamin D3 production? Physiol Biochem Zool 2003;76:52–9.

34. Gardiner DW, Baines FM, Pandher K. Photodermatitis and photokeratoconjunctivitis in a ball python (Python regius) and a blue-tongue skink (Tiliqua spp.). J Zoo Wildl Med 2009;40:757–66.

35. Young RJ. Environmental enrichment for captive animals. Oxford (United Kingdom): Blackwell Publishing; 2003.

36. Mellen JD, McPhee MS. Philosophy of environmental enrichment: past, present, and future. Zoo Biol 2001;20:211–26.

37. Blake E, Sherriff D, Skelton T. Environmental enrichment of reptiles. In: Afield D, editor. Guidelines for environmental enrichment: world zoo conservation strategy. West Sussex (United Kingdom): Association of British Wild Animal Keepers; 1998. p. 43–9.

38. Burghardt GM. Environmental enrichment and cognitive complexity in reptiles and amphibians: concepts, review, and implications for captive populations. Appl Anim Behav Sci 2013;147:286–98.

39. Davis KM, Burghardt GM. Training and long-term memory of a novel food acquisition task in a turtle (Pseudemys nelsoni). Behav Processes 2007;75:225–30.

40. Almli LM, Burghardt GM. Environmental enrichment alters the behavioral profile of rat snakes (Elaphe). J Appl Anim Welf Sci 2006;9:85–109.

41. Phillips CJ, Jiang Z, Hatton AJ, et al. Environmental enrichment for captive Eastern blue-tongue lizards (Tiliqua scincoides). Anim Welf 2011;20:377–84.

42. Burghardt GM, Ward B, Rosscoe R. Problem of reptile play: environmental enrichment and play behavior in a captive Nile softshell turtle, Trionyx triunguis. Zoo Biol 1996;15:223–38.

43. Kellerhouse K, Chepko-Sade D, Porter N. A slow-release cricket feeder tube decreases aggression and increases foraging in a mixed species exhibit of desert lizards (Iguanidae). Proceedings of the International Conference on Environmental Enrichment. New York: 2005. p. 217.

44. Hellmuth H, Augustine L, Watkins B, et al. Use of operant conditioning and desensitization to facilitate veterinary care with captive reptiles. Vet Clin North Am Exot Anim Pract 2012;15:425–43.

45. Fleming GJ. The use of operant conditioning in crocs. Proceedings of the North American Veterinary Conference. Orlando (FL): 2007. p. 1538.

46. Marlena D, Lafebre S. Moving the giants! Operant conditioning of Aldabra tortoises (Aldabrachelys [Geochelone] gigantea) to facilitate transfer to a new exhibit. Proceedings of the International Conference on Environmental Enrichment. Vienna (Austria): 2007. p. 109–12.

47. Weiss E, Wilson S. The use of classical and operant conditioning in training Aldabra tortoises (Aldabrachelys [Geochelone] gigantea) for venipuncture and other husbandry issues. J Appl Anim Welf Sci 2013;6:33–8.

48. Ethier N, Balsamo C. Training sea turtles for husbandry and enrichment. Proceedings of the International Conference on Environmental Enrichment. New York: 2005. p. 106–10.
49. Elsey RM, Joanen T, McNease L, et al. Growth rate and plasma corticosterone levels in juvenile alligators maintained at different stocking densities. J Exp Zool 1990;255:30–6.
50. Finke MD. Complete nutrient composition of commercially raised invertebrates used as food for insectivores. Zoo Biol 2002;21:269–85.
51. Oonincx DG, Dierenfeld ES. An investigation into the chemical composition of alternative invertebrate prey. Zoo Biol 2012;31:40–54.

Environmental Enrichment for Aquatic Animals

Mike Corcoran, DVM, CertAqV[a,b,c,]*

KEYWORDS

- Fish enrichment • Fish medicine • Aquatic animal enrichment • Koi enrichment
- Tropical fish enrichment • Aquarium enrichment • Octopus enrichment

KEY POINTS

- Enrichment decreases stress in captive animals and helps to promote natural behaviors.
- Effective enrichment programs decrease stereotypies and other abnormal behaviors.
- The basis for proper enrichment is proper husbandry, which includes excellent water quality when discussing aquatic animals.
- Enrichment varies by species, age, and must sometimes be tailored individually.
- Training animals for medical procedures increases the effectiveness of medical treatment and decreases the associated risks for the animal and the staff.

AN ARGUMENT FOR ENRICHMENT IN FISH

The need for enrichment in captive animals is based on the fact that animals are capable of experiencing pain, stress, and boredom. There are a number of peer-reviewed journal articles published even in recent decades that question these abilities in fish. As such, this author feels that it is important to highlight some of the more recent publications and research debunking those old concepts so that readers have the more current information at hand.

Several arguments have been presented against the idea that fish have consciousness or the ability to experience pain and suffering. The basis for these arguments was the absence of a neocortex in fish. The assumption is that the neocortex is the center of consciousness, and animals without a neocortex (such as fish) are unable to experience consciousness and, therefore, do not experience pain or suffering.[1] More recent work has shown this to be an oversimplified approach to the issue. Consciousness has been linked with the thalamocortical system and is generated by a complex neural

There are no conflicts of interest to report.
[a] VCA Wakefield Animal Hospital, 19 Main Street, Wakefield, MA 01880, USA; [b] American Association of Fish Veterinarians, 4580 Crackersport Road, Allentown, PA 18104, USA; [c] World Aquatic Veterinary Medical Association, 132 Lichfield Road, Stafford, Staffordshire ST17 4LE, UK
* VCA Wakefield Animal Hospital, 19 Main Street, Wakefield, MA 01880.
E-mail address: mike.corcoran@vca.com

process rather than in a single region of the brain.[2] In humans, the limbic system is the only area that consistently responds during perception of pain in imaging studies.[2] Anatomically, both A-delta and C fibers, which transmit pain, have been identified in the trigeminal nerves of fish. Stimulation of these nerves has been shown to stimulate areas of the brain involved in learning and emotion.[2–4] The brains of teleost fish develop differently than mammalian brains. During embryologic development, the neural tube folds outward in fish, and inward in mammals. However, there are homologous areas of the fish brain corresponding with the hippocampus and amygdala in mammals, where emotion and learning take place.[4] Comparing brain development, very conservative evolution has been observed among all vertebrates, with relatively similar brain function.[4] Advances in the understanding of neuroanatomy and neurophysiology support the idea that fish are able to develop consciousness and experience pain.

A second argument presented theorizes that, although aquatic animals respond to painful stimuli, they only react in a reflexive manner, with no understanding of the implications or emotional experience in association with the stimulus. Numerous studies have contradicted this theory. Trout injected with either acetic acid or bee venom had a significantly prolonged time approaching food compared with controls injected with saline. They also showed increased opercular movement and many rubbed the injection site on the substrate. All of these changes were mediated when fish were given an injection of morphine before the noxious stimulus.[4] Another study demonstrated that trout and goldfish both learned to avoid a specific region of a tank when that area was associated with an electrical shock. Interestingly, trout elected to remain in that region of the tank and be subjected to low-level electrical shocks when a conspecific was visible on that end of the tank. Goldfish remained near the middle of the tank when a conspecific was presented rather than retreating to the opposite end of the tank.[5] Both of these studies showed a clear difference in behavior based on a noxious stimulus. There was reduction of approach to a desired reward (food) or willingness to tolerate a noxious stimulus if offered socialization. Additionally, there was recognition of the specific area of stimulation and an attempt to relieve discomfort by rubbing. This is not limited to fish. A study involving hermit crabs had similar results. The crabs were placed into 2 different types of shells. Previous studies demonstrated a preference of one over the other for hermit crabs. When an electrical shock was applied to the crabs, there was a significant difference in the likelihood of the crab evacuating the shell. Far more evacuated the less desirable shell compared with the other type. There were also observed acts of shock-related aggression toward the evacuated shell.[6] Even if these studies do not clearly prove an emotional and conscious perception of pain in aquatic animals, they do demonstrate behavior responses beyond reflexive withdrawal in response to noxious stimuli. This evidence should justify the need for minimizing pain for these animals.

There has also been evidence of stress and fear demonstrated in fish. Acute stress from capture has clearly been associated with elevated cortisol and glucose levels in fish.[3,7] Fear responses associated with imminent electrical shock in goldfish have been ameliorated with N-methyl-D-aspartate antagonists and fear responses associated with an alarm pheromone in fish have been ameliorated with benzodiazepine treatment.[3] Fish introduced to a novel environment show increased foraging behavior when treated with benzodiazepine medication.[3] Restraint of some fish for 3 minutes or more decreased a behavioral pain response to injection of formalin. The behavior change was reduced if fish were pretreated with naloxone, demonstrating that the behavior change was owing to endogenous opioids released during acute stress from restraint.[8] Studies in fish have demonstrated that subordinate fish experience chronic stress owing to the presence of dominant fish, regardless of the actual aggressive behavior.[3] Because one of the main objectives for enrichment is to alleviate stress and encourage natural behaviors, it should be justified by these observations.

The last argument to be presented in support of offering enrichment for fish addresses the memory of fish. Most readers have probably heard the myth that by the time a fish swims around its fish bowl that it has forgotten what it originally saw in the bowl. In the latter sections of this article, training is discussed. The studies and methods of training clearly show that fish are able to form long-term memories.

HUSBANDRY ASPECTS OF ENRICHMENT

Environmental enrichment can be defined in many ways. It commonly involves altering the living environment of captive animals to allow more natural behaviors, provide more stimulation and enhance the physiologic and psychological well-being of the animals.[9] It is often also based on the "5 freedoms" guidelines described for welfare of terrestrial farm animals (**Box 1**). It is easy to see that ensuring proper husbandry is the first step to achieving these goals. For aquatic animals, this includes nutrition, housing, lighting, substrate, temperature, filtration, and water quality.

Nutrition

Nutrition for fish is complicated. Much of the research is focused on production fish rather than ornamental fish, but much information can be extrapolated from that research and applied to ornamental species. For a recent review of aquatic animal nutrition, see the September 2014 issue of *Veterinary Clinics of North America*.

Generally, protein levels should be 25% to 55% of the diet, depending on the species.[10–13] The protein source should be primarily animal proteins; fish meal is best.[12] Essential amino acids in fish are similar to those of other species, although arginine is far more important for fish than for mammals.[10,11] Fats should constitute 15% to 25% of the diet and fish require n-3 fatty acids.[13] Fish oils are the best source for the required fatty acids, and in general vegetable oils are a poor nutritional source for aquatic animals.[14] Carbohydrates are far less important to fish than to mammals. Starches are more digestible than sugars and should make up about 10% of the diet.[14] Most aquatic animal diets provide the needed vitamins so long as the diet is properly stored. The foods should be protected from heat, light, and moisture and be used within 6 months. Minerals are usually provided by the water directly and do not require supplementation in the diet if water quality is good.[10,13,14] See **Fig. 1** for general ratios of elements in the diet.

With respect to enrichment, there are a number of options involving foods. The specific diets for specific animals does require some knowledge of the species, at least the type of environment it has in the wild and whether it is a carnivore, omnivore or herbivore. Beyond that, some degree of variety is good for most species of aquatic

---

Box 1
Five freedoms of welfare for terrestrial farm animals (Farm Animal Welfare Council)

1. Freedom from hunger and thirst

2. Freedom from discomfort

3. Freedom from pain, injury, or disease

4. Freedom to express normal behavior

5. Freedom from fear and distress

Omnivorous and Herbivorous Fish

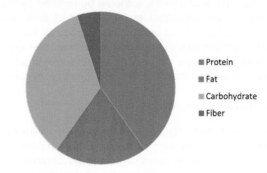

Carnivorous Fish

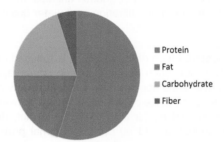

Fig. 1. Nutritional recommendations for fish.

animals. Again, there is not the degree of dietary knowledge for ornamental fish compared with that available for other domestic species. Offering a variety of foods within the general guidelines above can help to ensure that all nutrients are offered. Any nutrients missing from one diet can be made up for with others. Until long term nutritional studies can be performed on ornamental fish, this offers the best option for nutritional well-being. Keep in mind that many ornamental fish are still wild caught animals or 1–2 generations of captive breeding, so they do not have generations of selective breeding adapting them to conditions in captivity. While many canines and felines do not tolerate variation in diet, wild fish normally have a great deal of variety in their diets (depending on the species).

Variations in the diet also offer novel stimulation for psychological well-being. Commercial fish diets come in a wide range of formulations: live food, liquid diets, frozen diets, flakes, pellets, and gels. Among these there are also variations in size, shape, and color. Pellets can either be formulated to float at the surface or sink to the substrate. Some of the diets have full prey items like Mysis shrimp. Each of these has the potential to offer novelty when rotated. Live foods have the potential to introduce disease and parasites, and some of the diet formulations are not appropriate for all species. Knowledge of the species in a system as well as other aspects of filtration and husbandry helps to guide the choices offered to each animal.

Feeding Behavior

As with any enrichment, the natural behavior of the animal needs to be considered when selecting feeding enrichment. Different species of fish may feed by scavenging, foraging, grazing, or hunting.[15] Learning these normal behaviors for the fish being cared for helps to guide an enrichment program and helps to evaluate the success of the selected program. In addition to changing the type of food offered, other changes can help to keep feeding novel. Some methods that have been implemented successfully include a rotation in feeding times and locations. Currents being added at feeding times can simulate hunting with prekilled food.[15] Sea horses have been fed with sinking canisters of brine shrimp and with frozen sinking cubes of shrimp. Increased foraging behavior was seen with both strategies.[15,16] Foraging has also been encouraged by sinking feeders with holes. The feeders are filled with live feed that slowly disperse from the feeder.[15] Animals that prefer to hide (eels, gobis, etc) may need to be focus fed with sinking food placed by a dropper or by feeding with tongs. Submissive fish should have special attention during feedings to ensure they are getting adequate nutrition (**Fig. 2**).[12]

The last part of any nutritional enrichment program is monitoring. The caretaker should watch the fish for natural behaviors, and the amount of time spent in feeding behaviors. Body condition of animals should also be monitored regularly. If any decreased activity or weight loss is observed, the program should be reevaluated and, in the case of weight loss, a medical evaluation should be considered.

Housing

For aquatic animals, we are of course discussing either a bowl, aquarium, or pond. Much is in common between the 15 gallon aquarium in a home and the 15,000 gallon aquarium at a zoo. Both require the size to be appropriate for the species held, the proper current, filtration, lighting, substrate, depth, and dimensions.

Size is the first important consideration when considering what animals can be placed in an enclosure (or what enclosure is appropriate for a certain animal to be displayed). Size considerations include not only length and width, but depth and volume. Dimensions in the tank (length, width, and depth) are extremely important for some species and less important for others. Knowledge of the species is important for these decisions and proper dimensions are necessary for the animal to be able to display natural behaviors, and to have freedom from stress and discomfort. Several examples are highlighted to help the reader begin to learn what considerations are necessary in either tank design or deciding whether or not a certain species can have proper enrichment in an existing system.

One good example on a large scale is preparation and selection of appropriate aquarium space for sharks. Many sharks are pelagic and obligate ram breathers. *Pelagic*

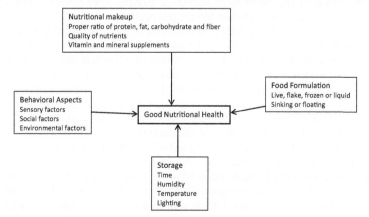

Fig. 2. Aspects of nutritional health for aquatic animals.

means they are more commonly found in open water away from shore and off the bottom. *Obligate ram breathers* means they must continue moving forward to get adequate water flow across their gills for proper respiration.[17] To conserve energy, these sharks move forward with a long gliding phase to their swimming pattern, utilizing their pectoral fins to generate lift and conserve energy. If the enclosure is too short, more energy is required for movement, and not only do the animals become exhausted, but natural swimming behavior is restricted. There are formulaic guidelines for determining dimensions, but shape of the aquarium and location of obstructions to movement (such as reefs) can affect the formulas and must be considered.[17,18] Overhead clearance in most of these aquariums also needs to allow unobstructed movement for dorsal fins out of the water.[18]

Depth can be important for certain species as well. Some marine fish are accustomed to living on reefs with steep vertical walls. One factor regarding depth can be light penetration through water. Water is a powerful filter of light. Red light penetrates a very short distance and the blue end of the visible light spectrum is filtered deeper. Coral depends on certain wavelengths of light to get energy from photosynthesis from the symbiotic zooxanthellae.[19] The depth of the water and placement of lighting has a profound effect on the health of these animals.

Depth may also be a factor in design based on the function and purpose of the aquarium with consideration for the health of the animals on display. Dimensions of touch tanks vary from those of tanks purely for display. A relatively shallow depth ensures easier interaction for visitors at a public aquarium. It also reduces surface area of skin from visitors when they reach into the water. This decreases toxin exposure for aquatic animals from hand lotions and skin bacteria. It also decreases visitor's exposure to zoonotic diseases.[20] The horizontal size of display tanks needs to ensure adequate space for the animals on display and should give the ability for the animals to have choice in interaction with visitors, but allow them to distance themselves from handling as well.[18] If it is not possible to allow choice (eg, starfish that move too slowly), then 2 tanks should be used in alternating fashion or an off-display holding tank should allow rotation of animals.[20]

Proper current is the next consideration to be discussed after the size of the tank. Proper water flow in a system is also heavily species dependent. Betta fish have very large fins and naturally inhabit stagnant water in rice patties of Asia. Even a very light current in a system can be very stressful or even harmful for them. On the opposite extreme, very high flow rates are required for some systems containing river fish. Salmon ladders built into dams allow salmon to bypass. They need to have a strong current to ensure that salmon follow the proper route upstream. In the middle, coral require some current to carry food and nutrients to them because they are largely stationary in a system, but too strong of a current can damage their fragile appendages.[21] Proper water flow in a system also affects aeration and filtration of the water. Betta fish are labyrinth fish, meaning they can breathe air at the surface. They are also tolerant of poor water quality relative to other species, so low water flow is fine as long as the water changes are frequent enough. By contrast, some marine species have greater oxygen requirements. Salt water also has less holding capacity for oxygen. If the water flow is interrupted in a tropical salt water tank, some species of fish suffocate within hours. Koi ponds are normally designed with waterfalls or fountains, not only for decoration, but for aeration of the water as well. Without this aeration, water in these ponds can be oxygen depleted and can have increased waste gasses.[22] For enrichment, some water flow can be changed with the right species of fish. Most filtration systems have movable spouts to direct the flow of water leaving the filter and returning to the aquarium. There are also underwater fans or jets that attach to the inside of the aquarium and can be located in different areas of the tank easily. It is relatively simple to create a tidal motion using a reservoir at one end of an enclosure that gradually fills and then rapidly empties water returning to the aquarium from the filtration system. Tidal action is frequently used in public aquariums in the touch tanks, often filtering down through various shallow pools of different levels. Many touch tank animals (starfish, small crabs, etc) live in tidal pools and do well with this type of enrichment.

The next consideration in the system is the substrate and decorations placed in the tank. All the contents in the aquarium or pond can offer some enrichment. Substrate can vary in color, size, and texture. They can look natural or very artificial, from sand to colored glass beads. Although they are designed to present different decorative effects for the observer in most cases, they are also important for the fish. They can be important for some spawning behavior, territory marking, and nest building.[9] Some examples help to illustrate the importance of ensuring the substrate is proper for the species. Southern stingrays are accustomed to burying themselves in the sand. They should be offered a fine, nonabrasive sand deep enough to bury themselves. Garden eels need a mix of fine sand and crushed coral 8 to 12 inches deep to allow them to burrow to be free from fear and anxiety.[23]

The number and type of decorations available is almost without limit. Just like substrate, they can be very natural in material or appearance or can be very artificial. Different options include rocks, plants (real and artificial), PVC pipes, wood, statues, and mechanical toys. Rocks can provide a natural appearance to the environment and add a vertical dimension to the enclosure. When arranged properly, they can also form caves and provide hiding places for inhabitants that feel more comfortable in caves or crevices.[9] The increased surface area can provide more biological filtration in the system (discussed further in the sections on filtration and water quality elsewhere in this article). PVC pipes can be hidden under the rocks or holes can be drilled into the rocks to provide cave areas. Plants can also add a vertical component and a more natural appearance to the environment. They can provide shade to outdoor pond fish. Wood can be a source of nutrients to some snails in aquariums. The statues and mechanical toys like Tiki heads, skulls, "bubble volcanoes," and treasure chests are largely decorative, but can still provide hiding places for submissive fish and novel items for exploration. Even providing these items and rotating them randomly can change daily patterns and provide new territory.[9,15]

Lighting

Many advances in lighting offer great options for enrichment. Different lighting can enhance the experiences of the observer and can enhance the well-being of the inhabitants or the system. Specific lighting can even be important for growth and breeding with some species. Starting with coral, the importance of lighting spectrum can be emphasized. Coral depend on nutrients from their zooxanthellae for growth. The blue end of the visible light spectrum is the best for photosynthesis by these organisms and is associated with the best coral growth. By contrast, red lighting has been associated with coral bleaching events.[21] Variation can also be provided by length of day. The standard beginning photoperiod is 12 hours each of dark and light, but this cycle rarely occurs for fish in the wild. Varying day length has been implicated in the breeding cycles and other behaviors in many species of fish that are seasonal breeders or that have seasonal migrations.[24]

Various types of lighting are also available for aquariums. Fluorescent lighting is common and bulbs are available with focuses of different wavelengths for different purposes. Metal halide lighting offers more intense lighting that also seems to be more natural in the aquarium.[21] More recently, LED lighting has been introduced to aquarium lighting systems. The cost of these systems is now coming down to a point that they are becoming practical for even hobbyists to have access. Not only do LED systems offer better penetration into the water column, but they allow other features that are great for enrichment. New systems are programmable. The day length can be adjusted automatically throughout the year. The lights can also better simulate natural lighting by gradually dimming at the end of the day and reversing in the morning to simulate sunrise and sunset. Because LED systems are designed with multiple smaller lights, cloud cover and thunderstorm effects are available with some systems. The effects of this enrichment on fish behavior is a good subject for future research. It can be proposed that providing more natural lighting effects will have a positive effect on promoting natural behaviors in aquarium inhabitants.

FILTRATION AND WATER QUALITY

There are no unique aspects of filtration or water quality that provide novel experiences for enrichment, but discussing aspects of husbandry that promote natural behavior, physical health, and psychological health should include these topics with regard to aquatic animals. In most natural environments, there is a tremendous turnover of water that keeps contaminants from accumulating. In a closed pond or aquarium, animals live in the same water in which they eat and eliminate waste. Without proper water quality, natural behaviors cannot occur and there is greater chance of disease and stress.

Filtration

Filtration for aquatic systems comes in 3 different types: mechanical, chemical and biological.[22,25] Most systems use a combination of at least 2 of these types of filtration. Mechanical filtration uses different methods to physically remove material from the water. The filters may use sand, gravel, felt cloth, or other material to strain large suspended material from the water. Mechanical filtration contributes to the clarity of the water in a system, but can also help to prevent buildup of nitrogenous waste by removing large particles of food or other biological material from the water before decomposition. For these filters to work properly, they require some routine maintenance. The material may need to be replaced or the filter may require that the material is stirred to avoid formation of channels that bypass the bulk of the material.

Chemical filtration uses chemical reactions to remove dissolved substances from the water.[22] The most common use of chemical filtration is use of a dechlorinating agent to prepare water. It is important to note that most city water systems now contain chloramines, a more stable form of chlorine. Conventional wisdom is that chlorine evaporates from water in 24 hours, but this is not true of chloramines. If a chemical dechlorinator is not used, then toxicity from chlorine is likely to result from using the water. Other examples of chemical filtration include activated charcoal, foam fractionation, UV sterilization, and ozonation.[22,25,26] Activated charcoal is used in fresh water and marine systems to remove ammonia, medications, or and some heavy metals. Foam fractionation is used primarily in marine systems. Very fine bubbles are formed in a closed container. The hydrophobic end of proteins is trapped in the bubbles and elevated to a collection cup at the top of the water column.[22,26] UV sterilization is used to irradiate the DNA and RNA of bacteria, viruses, algae, fungi, and protozoa. The UV light is placed in the pipes in an area of low flow to allow contact time.[22] Ozonation is generally used in larger systems. Ozone is produced in a closed container and exposed to the water. The ozone oxidizes organic compounds in the water.[22,25,26]

Biological filtration is present in almost all healthy systems. Organic material in the water breaks down quickly to ammonia. This material comes from feces, uneaten food, and dead animals or plants. Ammonia is toxic to fish and invertebrates. The biological filter consists of *Nitrosomonas* and *Nitrobacter* bacteria.[25] They break down the ammonia stepwise into nitrite and nitrate. This process is known as the nitrogen cycle (**Fig. 3**). Each step in the process is less toxic to the inhabitants of the aquarium. Nitrates can be removed either through periodic water changes or by conversion to nitrogen, which leaves the water as a gas.[22,25–27] To establish and maintain a biological filter, surface area must be provided to allow growth of bacteria. Various methods are used in different systems. Live rock and live sand can be used in plain sight on display for a natural appearance. Inside the filtration system, surface area can be provided by sponges, wheels, brushes, or plastic balls.

There are certain aspects of filtration that are also important to note for veterinarians and caretakers who would be involved in medical treatment. First, it is important to remember that chemical filtration is designed to remove contaminants based on chemical properties or chemical reactions. When adding medications to the water for treatment of sick fish, chemical filtration in the system needs to be considered. The same processes that remove toxins and proteins can also remove or inactivate medications. Depending on the treatment, chemical filtration may need to be discontinued temporarily.[28] This lapse can affect water quality, adding stress to animals that are already affected by infection or another stressor. Maintaining all other aspects of husbandry as close to normal is an important consideration for treatment. Second, biological filtration can be affected by some medical treatments. If the treatment kills the bacteria in the biological filter, poor water quality can result and the filter may need to be re-established after treatment. The poorer water quality will cause more stress to be added to the illness in the fish. Finally, activated charcoal has been highly correlated with head and lateral line erosion, a disease that may cause an animal to be presented to a veterinarian.[29] The caretaker or practitioner should consider the effect of antibiotics or other

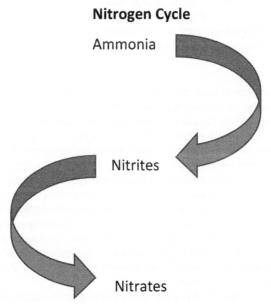

Nitrogen Cycle

Ammonia

Nitrites

Nitrates

Fig. 3. The nitrogen cycle.

medications on the bacteria of the biological filter.[28] This will also add stress to the animals under treatment. Any enrichment that can reduce the stresses associated with treatment will help to maintain good health. Training animals for medical procedures is discussed elsewhere as an important method for stress reduction.

Water Quality

Monitoring and maintaining good water quality is among the most important aspects of aquatic animal care and enrichment. If water quality is not adequate, then the animal cannot be free from discomfort or disease and cannot exhibit normal behaviors. No matter the type of system, the caretaker should monitor and maintain normal ammonia, nitrites, nitrates, temperature, pH, and alkalinity. Other parameters that may need to be maintained in various systems include total hardness, salinity, dissolved oxygen, calcium, copper, magnesium, oxidation reduction potential, phosphate, and dissolved organic material, among others. The brevity of this section is not a reflection of the importance of water quality maintenance in an enrichment program; rather, the opposite is true. Entire books have been written on the subject of water quality. There is no way possible to have an inclusive section in this article that would adequately address water quality for enrichment. The reader who is unfamiliar with water quality should make an effort to learn as much as possible on the subject.

ENRICHMENT BASED ON LIFE STAGES
Fish Fry

Fish fry (newborns, not food) should be separated immediately from adults in most cases. Infanticide is common with many aquatic animals in captivity. Husbandry varies by species, but in most cases the fry need to be protected from high water flow. This is usually done by placing the fry in a refugium inside the aquarium so that there is some water flow, but less than the normal aquarium. Water quality parameters, temperature, and light cycles should be determined on a species-specific basis. Generally, larval fish require live food for survival. In 1 study, fish larvae raised initially on dry food showed 100% mortality by 15 days compared with 100% survival in larvae raised on live food up to 15 mg of weight.[30] Live food has the advantage of stimulating natural behavior in fish and may offer enrichment. The drawback is the potential for introduction of parasites or disease.

Quarantine

Newly acquired fish should always be held in strict quarantine. The author recommends a time period between 30 and 90 days depending on the species, water temperature, and source of acquisition. Quarantine also presents some unique enrichment challenges. A normal quarantine enclosure has scant material in the aquarium or pond. Any substrate, live rock, or other porous surfaces are not easily disinfected between acquired animals. Excessive hiding areas make close observation of quarantined animals difficult. Porous materials can also interfere with prophylactic medications used in quarantine. This difficulty necessitates a more artificial environment that is devoid of much of the normal enrichment. At the same time, it can be a period of greatly increased stress for the animals. Often, animals have been shipped over long distances just before quarantine. Many are recently wild caught and are unaccustomed to an aquarium. During quarantine in many facilities, animals are subject to medications, sedation, and multiple examinations that add to the stress. Any allowances for reduced stress improves the survivability of quarantined animals.

When possible, animals should be allowed several days to acclimate to the new surroundings before starting prophylactic treatments or performing examinations. In many cases, feeding animals is inappropriate for the first several days of quarantine. PVC pipe or other similar material can be placed into the quarantine tanks to provide hiding areas for fish and reduce stress.[31] Water quality should be maintained strictly. Temperature should be maintained within the normal parameters. Many advocate maintaining the temperature at the high end of normal to accelerate parasite life cycles, but this needs to be balanced with stress to the animals. It is safer to use normal temperatures and extend the time in quarantine. Stocking density should be low in quarantine to reduce stress on the animals in the systems.[31] Quarantine is also not a safe area to mix predators with their prey items, although this is sometimes done on display in larger systems with adequate hiding spaces for the prey animals. Examples are large capacity reef aquariums that house sharks with other fish species to display all animals present in the ecosystem. Lighting should reflect normal spectrum and timing for the species and nutrition should be high quality.

Display

For the purpose of this article, display tanks are the systems in which the animals are maintained on a long-term or permanent basis. Display tanks can be extremely different when looking across all possibilities. Home hobby aquariums, backyard ponds, food farming facilities, and public educational aquariums all must be considered. Although there are many differences, some basic principles apply to all. First, the size of the aquarium determines the species that can be displayed (or the desired species determines the size of the enclosure needed). The species kept in the system determines the remainder of the husbandry. Every effort should be made to keep only species from the same regions of the world. Husbandry varies for fresh water fish from the Amazon and Asian river, as it will between marine fish from the Pacific and the Caribbean. The species selected (or already present in a system newly assigned) determine the water quality parameters and water temperature. It also determines the necessary lighting, water flow, filtration, substrate depth, and dietary needs. Once husbandry needs have been met, further enrichment can be established.

Again, the goal of enrichment is to encourage natural behaviors. In nature there is no feeding schedule, but in captivity it is necessary to have some type of schedule so that food intake can be monitored and so that excess food does not adversely affect water quality. In nature, excess ammonia is diluted in large bodies of water. In captivity, stocking density is much higher than in the wild, so waste is far more concentrated. With these limitations, adjustments must be made to normal feeding, but the changes can be mediated with an enrichment program. Just like other animals, the time spent engaged in hunting or foraging in the wild is far more than captive animals on a feeding schedule. It is well-documented in most other animals that the resulting time, if unoccupied, leads to stereotypies and other abnormal behaviors. To deter these problems, foraging programs are established. The same enrichment can be adjusted to captive aquatic animals. With most aquatic animals, the actual diet can be varied. Offering different foods can be enriching and can also help to ensure better food intake and good nutritional balance.[9] The feeding schedule and location of feeding stations can also be varied to prevent entrainment to particular foods and schedules.[9,15] Feeding near currents can stimulate hunting behavior by forcing fish to swim after the food.[15] Multiple daily feedings also helps to simulate a more natural feeding regime. For herbivorous or omnivorous species, plants in the enclosure allow grazing throughout the day. Finally, foraging devices can be formed by drilling holes in closed canisters and filling with brine shrimp or other food.[15]

Lighting changes can be an integral part of an enrichment program. Natural sunlight does not turn on and off with a switch. The wavelength and intensity of light is again dictated by the tank design and the species on display. Enrichment can be built into the design by varying the lighting. Rather than an instant on and off, lighting can be programmed to go on and off more gradually to simulate sunrise and sunset. At the most simple, various lights are created for different wavelengths of light. The Actinic blue bulbs can be turned on earlier than the full spectrum in the morning and left on longer in the evening. However, with newer LED lighting systems, the lights can be preprogrammed to go on and off like a dimmer. These systems can also allow seasonal variations in day length. Cloud cover and storms can be simulated on some of the more advanced LED systems or with changing the intensity of other lights. Night lighting can be provided to simulate moonlight and this can also be altered to simulate monthly variation in intensity.[9]

Furnishings need to be selected based on the species and natural behaviors. Many aquatic animals require hiding areas to be free from fear and distress; others need unobstructed access to lighting for proper nutrition. Various substrates, rock formations, PVC piping, and other sculptures are available for home hobbyists and public aquariums alike. Periodic changes to furnishings can be integrated into a foraging program. Most aquatic animals move to new environments in the course of their normal interaction. Even if living on the same reef, fish move to new areas periodically in search of food, mates, or new shelter. Changes to furnishings can reflect seasonal changes of the natural environment of some species.[15] Rearranging existing furnishings periodically can also encourage animals to seek new territory and explore the enclosure more thoroughly. Novel furnishings provide opportunities to explore and defend as new territory.[15] Keep in mind there are some species that do not normally experience novel environments as often. For example, Betta fish inhabit small niche areas in the wild. For these species, excessive change can be stressful as well. Knowing as much as possible about the natural environment of the species is important as a foundation for development of an enrichment program.

Water movement needs vary with species.[9] From one extreme to the other, some fish require a very stagnant enclosure, whereas others live in tidal regions that have regular, drastic changes to flow. Most aquariums and ponds have external filtration. Placement of the inflow and outflow of the filtration establishes the basal water movement in the system. The number, location, and diameter of these pipes can change the water flow pattern in a system. In many aquariums, they are locked in place by designs; in others, they can be changed. In addition to the flow established by filtration, water flow can be changed with supplemental equipment. Underwater fans can be attached to the inside of aquarium glass and used to direct the flow of water (**Fig. 4**). These fans can be rearranged regularly to change water flow. There are also systems that allow rapid water changes like what is found in a tidal pool. The outflow of the filtration system fills a container to a certain level, then the container empties rapidly, providing high flow into the system. These systems can be created with spring-loaded buckets that dump when filled or more elaborate systems with a mechanism similar to toilet flappers.

Training for Medical Procedures

Training programs are established for many species of animals to accept medical treatment voluntarily. This training reduces the need for anesthesia and stressful capturing. Trained animals demonstrate reduced cortisol levels during medical procedures when compared with control animals.[32] Target training has been successful in many varied species of aquatic animals.[33–36] This training is the first step in training for medical procedures. The target can be a colored panel, light, or any other object readily identifiable by the animal that is not permanently in place inside the enclosure.

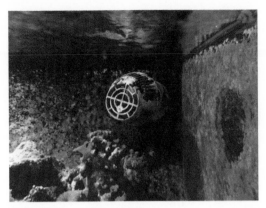

Fig. 4. Circulating pump used to create current.

Contact with the target is bridged with a reward, usually a food item. The food item can be attached to the target or given by a caretaker upon contact with the target. The animal is then trained to target for varying lengths of time to get the reward.[33] Once the target training is established, then bridging that training with other procedures can be started. Target training alone can be used to separate various animals. At the New York Aquarium, aggressive sharks were targeted to 1 side of an enclosure and sea turtles were targeted to the other side for treatment.[34] Target training can also be used to target animals into treatment tanks in large enclosures to decrease capture stress.[34,36]

Target training can also be used for specific procedures. Animals can be asked to go to their targets in association with a stretcher, net, or other capture device in proximity to the target. The capture device is placed in front of the target, deep to the animal. As the animal is desensitized to the presence of the net, it can gradually be brought closer until the animal accepts voluntary capture for weight checks or transport.[33,34,36] Common medical procedures that can also be associated with target training include skin scrapes, ultrasound examination, medication administration, phlebotomy, and handling for examination of the ventral aspect of the animal. Similar methods are used as for capture. While the animal is targeted, tactile stimulation is coupled with the reward. As the animal is desensitized to the touch, it can be increased gradually until the animal accepts injections, phlebotomy, ultrasound probe contact, or handling for examination.[36] Some degree of training in this manner has been performed on sharks, rays, and even goldfish. Acceptance of any of these procedures voluntarily decreases stress and risk associated with procedures (**Fig. 5**).

ENRICHMENT FOR SPECIFIC ANIMALS
Koi

Koi are among the most popular aquatic animals seen by veterinarians in private practice. With their long lifespan and high monetary value, some are seen on a regular basis for routine health care or chronic medical concerns. Enrichment recommendations can be a valuable part of that care. The author discusses some rotation of feeding schedules and multiple small feedings throughout the day. Plants in the pond should be placed in a way that offers shade and cover from predators. The plants can be rotated periodically for enrichment.

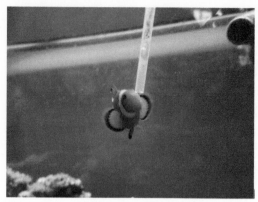

Fig. 5. The author's fish, Krusty, targeting to a food pipette.

Owners can also be encouraged to do some target training and can do some training for voluntary medical procedures. Koi are extremely food motivated and readily respond to the appearance of their caretakers (and in personal experience the presence of the veterinarian). They are intelligent and willing to learn. The methods described herein can be used easily with koi to train them for low-stress capture and get them accustomed to handling. The author has been able to perform ultrasound, skin scrapes, injections, orogastric intubation, and even phlebotomy on some koi without sedation.

Elasmobranchs

Sharks and rays are common animals to appear in collections at public aquariums and are seen occasionally in private collections. They are also intelligent and readily trained. Not only will training for procedures and handling reduce their stress, but it is important to remember that many of these animals can pose a threat to the caretakers. Training can reduce the need for direct handling for many procedures and can allow easier safe restraint. Reduced stress for the animal at procedure times also decreases the chances that the animal shows defensive behaviors, such as biting or stinging.

Cephalopods

Octopuses are some of the most popular animals at public aquariums. Their intelligence has been recognized for some time and enrichment has been well-documented for the giant pacific octopus (GPO). GPOs kept in captivity without aggressive enrichment programs frequently display inking, irregular color patterns, jetting into the sides of the enclosure, and autophagy.[37] They are also notorious escape artists. The escape attempts can be dangerous to the octopuses as well as inhabitants of nearby enclosures; they have been known to hunt in adjacent enclosures. Escape attempts were found to be far less frequent from tanks that had viewing windows as a form of environmental enrichment.[38] The author has personal knowledge of a GPO intentionally obstructing the drain to overflow its enclosure on days when a particular caretaker was absent. Enriched octopuses also had decreased periods of rest and explored a greater percentage of the enclosure.[37]

Multiple forms of enrichment have been documented in octopuses. One of the most simple and yet most effective is feeding live food.[37–39] There are definite ethical implications to the introduction of live prey in a limited size enclosure with its predator.

Allowances for hiding areas should be used to minimize the stress for the prey item. This also increases the time spent for the GPO exhibiting predatory behavior. A single crab introduced into an enclosure can provide hours of enrichment for an octopus.[38] Interaction with the caretakers is also a simple form of enrichment that seems to be appreciated by the GPO and can offer several hours of enrichment.[39] Unfamiliar plants and shells can be offered, especially in sizes that allow them to be used as shelters.[37] Food can be offered in a frozen cube or a puzzle box. A Mr Potato Head toy with food hidden on the inside has been used in several aquariums.[38,39] Food placed in floating toy boats requires that the object be sunk to feed.[39] Learning and exploration seems to be both visual and tactile, so novel attempts at enrichment should take these factors into consideration for increased chances of success.[37] As a side note related to the visual acuity of GPOs, flash photography has been shown to be very stressful and should be forbidden to prevent fear and stress.

SUMMARY

Enrichment is not a new concept in animal care. Proper enrichment has been shown to decrease stereotypies, increase exploration of enclosures, and decrease rest periods. The 5 freedoms for welfare in terrestrial animals have been used frequently as a frame of reference for enrichment programs. Utilizing these freedoms, enrichment programs are designed to decrease stress, increase natural behaviors, and by decreasing stress, decrease injury and disease. Aquatic animals need enrichment just as other captive animals. There are unique challenges presented by the aquatic environments in which they are kept, but the basic principles remain the same.

REFERENCES

1. Rose JD. The neurobehavioral nature of fishes and the question of awareness and pain. Rev Fish Sci 2002;10:1–38.
2. Chandroo KP, Yue S, Moccia RD. An evaluation of current perspectives on consciousness and -pain in fishes. Fish Fish 2004;5:281–95.
3. Chandroo KP, Duncan IJ, Moccia RD. Can fish suffer? perspectives on sentience, pain, fear and stress. Appl Anim Behav Sci 2004;86:225–50.
4. Braithwaite VA, Boulcott P. Pain perception, aversion and fear in fish. Dis Aquat Org 2007;75:131–8.
5. Dunlop R, Millsopp S, Laming P. Avoidance learning in goldfish (Carassius auratus) and trout (Oncorthynchus mykiss) and implications for pain perception. Appl Anim Behav Sci 2006;97:255–71.
6. Elwwod RW, Appel M. Pain experience in hermit crabs? Anim Behav 2009;77: 1243–6.
7. Kubokawa K, Watanabe T, Yoshioka M, et al. Effects of acute stress on plasma cortisol, sex steroid hormone and glucose levels in male and female sockeye salmon during the breeding season. Aquaculture 1999;172:335–49.
8. Wolkers CP, Barbosa A Jr, Menescal-de-Oliveria L, et al. Stress induced antinociception in fish reversed by naloxone. PLoS One 2013;8:e71175.
9. Williams TD, Readman GD, Owen SF. Key issues concerning environmental enrichment for laboratory-held fish species. Lab Anim 2009;43:107–20.
10. Lovell RT. Nutrition of aquaculture species. J Anim Sci 1991;69:4193–200.
11. King JO. Fish nutrition. Vet Rec 1973;92:546–50.
12. Mayer J. Fish nutrition and related problems. Compend Contin Educ Vet 2012; 34:1–4.

13. Lall SP, Tibbits SM. Nutrition, feeding and behavior in fish. Vet Clin North Am Exot Anim Pract 2009;12:361–72.

14. Olivia-Teles A. Nutrition and health of aquaculture fish. J Fish Dis 2012;35:83–101.

15. Suggested guidelines for fishes enrichment. American Association of Zookeepers. Available at: https://www.aazk.org/wp-content/uploads/Suggested-Guidelines-for-Fishes-Enrichment.pdf. Accessed September 17, 2014.

16. Hale E, Chepko-Sade D, Porter N. Increased foraging time in lined seahorses (*Hippocampus Erectus*) by using feeding enrichment with slow release (frozen) cubes of mysis shrimp. Proceedings of the Seventh International Conference on Environmental Enrichment. 2005. p. 53.

17. Choromanski JM. Quarantine and isolation facilities for elasmobranchs: design and construction. In: Smith M, Warmolts D, Thoney D, et al, editors. Elasmobranch husbandry manual: captive care of sharks, rays and their relatives. Columbus (OH): Ohio Biological Survey; 2004. p. 43–51.

18. Powell DC. Design and construction of exhibits for elasmobranchs. In: Smith M, Warmolts D, Thoney D, et al, editors. Elasmobranch husbandry manual: captive care of sharks, rays and their relatives. Columbus (OH): Ohio Biological Survey; 2004. p. 53–67.

19. Borneman EH. Zooxanthellae. In: Borneman E, editor. Aquarium corals: selection, husbandry and natural history. Neptune City (NJ): TFH Publications; 2009. p. 47–55.

20. Lawler A. Touch tanks. Available at: http://www.aquarticles.com/articles/management/Lawler_Touch_Tanks.html. Accessed August 26, 2014.

21. Borneman EH. Husbandry: captive reef-keeping approaches and essentials. In: Borneman E, editor. Aquarium corals: selection, husbandry and natural history. Neptune City (NJ): TFH Publications; 2009. p. 323–41.

22. Saint-Erne N. Environmental management. In: Saint-Erne N, editor. Advanced koi care for veterinarians and professional koi keepers. Glendale (AZ): Erne Enterprises; 2010. p. 88–126.

23. Roman R. Aquarium fish: a detailed look at the home aquarium husbandry of the spotted garden Eel. Available at: http://www.advancedaquarist.com/2011/7/fish2. Accessed September 10, 2014.

24. Feist BE, Anderson JJ. Review of fish behavior relevant to fish guidance systems. Annual Report of Research from University of Washington School of Fisheries. Seattle (WA): University of Washington; 1991.

25. Mohan PJ, Aiken A. Water quality and life support systems for large elasmobranch exhibits. In: Smith M, Warmolts D, Thoney D, et al, editors. Elasmobranch husbandry manual: captive care of sharks, rays and their relatives. Columbus (OH): Ohio Biological Survey; 2004. p. 69–88.

26. Moe MA Jr. Filtration: mechanical, chemical, biological and sterilization. In: Moe MA Jr, editor. Marine aquarium handbook: beginning to breeder. Neptune City (NJ): TFH Publications; 2009. p. 60–89.

27. Brightwell CR. The marine nitrogen cycle. In: Brightwell CR, editor. Marine chemistry: a complete guide to water chemistry in marine aquariums. Neptune City (NJ): TFH Publications; 2007. p. 59–70.

28. Noga EJ. General concepts in therapy. In: Noga E, editor. Fish disease: diagnosis and treatment. 2nd edition. Ames (IA): Blackwell Publishing; 2010. p. 347–73.

29. Stamper MA, Kittell MM, Patel EE, et al. Effects of full-stream carbon filtration on the development of head and lateral line erosion syndrome (HLLES) in ocean surgeon. J Aquat Anim Health 2011;23(3):111–6.

30. Bambroo P. On the diet substitution and adaptation weight in carp *Cyprinus carpo* larvae. Indian J Sci Res 2012;3:133–6.

31. Noga EJ. Health management. In: Fish disease: diagnosis and treatment. 2nd edition. Ames (IA): Blackwell Publishing; 2010. p. 69–79.
32. Koban T, Donmoyer MG, Hammar A. Effects of positive reinforcement training on cortisol, hematology and cardiovascular parameters in cynomolgus macaques (*Macaca fascicularis*). Proceedings of the Seventh International Conference on Environmental Enrichment. 2005. p. 233.
33. Foerder P. Target training in barramundi fish (*Lates calcarifer*). Proceedings of the Seventh International Conference on Environmental Enrichment. 2005. p. 112–7.
34. Ethier N, Balsamo C. Training sea turtles for husbandry and enrichment. Proceedings of the Seventh International Conference on Environmental Enrichment. 2005. p. 106–11.
35. Clark E. Instrumental conditioning of lemon sharks. Science 1959;130:217–8.
36. Corwin AL. Training fish and aquatic invertebrates for husbandry and medical behaviors. Vet Clin North Am Exot Anim Pract 2012;15:455–67.
37. Brady M, Rehling M, Mueller J, et al. Giant pacific octopus behavior and enrichment. International Zoo News. Available at: http://www.zoonews.co.uk/IZN/380/IZN-380-octopus.html. Accessed September 17, 2014.
38. Anderson RC, Wood JB. Enrichment for giant pacific octopuses: happy as a clam? J Appl Anim Welfare Sci 2001;4(2):157–68.
39. Slater M, Buttling O. Giant pacific octopus husbandry manual. London: The British and Irish Association for Zoos and Aquariums; 2011.

Special Article

Advances in Exotic Mammal Clinical Therapeutics

Michelle G. Hawkins, VMD, DABVP (Avian)

KEYWORDS

- Analgesic • Antibacterial • Antifungal • Antiparasitic • Small mammal
- Therapeutics

Although it is important to stay informed of the current medications used in exotic mammal veterinary practice, new drug delivery approaches being evaluated for safety, efficacy, and welfare factors are just as noteworthy. Sustained-release formulations of commonly used drugs and different methods of drug administration allow the exotic mammal veterinarian to reduce the stress of treatment in diverse situations. A recent example in mice identified the effective use of voluntary ingestion of albendazole-infused honey when compared with the typical method of oral administration via gavage feeding.[1] Interactions can occur between vehicle and drugs with many different combinations; consequently, studies are certainly warranted regarding these potential reactions. However, newer studies have been published that provide the basis for exploring the use of different vehicles, frequency of dosing, and drug delivery techniques for various classes of drugs in small mammals. The goals of this article are to not only evaluate new medications or uses for medications in exotic mammal veterinary practice but also review new methods of drug delivery that might be useful to the exotic mammal practitioner.

THERAPEUTIC DELIVERY SYSTEMS

Bony infections, including dental abscesses, have provided significant challenges for exotic mammal practitioners as antibiotic penetration becomes a significant concern. Systemic antibiotic treatment occasionally needs to be supplemented with local antibiotic therapeutic delivery routes such as antibiotic-impregnated polymethylmethacralate beads,[2–5] antibiotic-impregnated gauze,[6] long-lasting doxycycline gel,[7] honey,[8] calcium hydroxide,[8,9] or bioactive ceramics.[2,10] Recently, newer hydrogels

This article originally appeared in Journal of *Exotic Pet Medicine*, Volume 23, Number 1, 2014.
Department of Medicine and Epidemiology, School of Veterinary Medicine, University of California-Davis, 2108 Tupper Hall, Davis, CA 95616, USA
E-mail address: mghawkins@ucdavis.edu

have been applied in stem cell therapy and cancer research.[11,12] These new hydrogels can facilitate controlled drug release. Moreover, the porous structure of the material and its affinity to its therapeutic payload can be chemically controlled without affecting inherent physicochemical compatibility to natural tissues.[11] Hydrogels are an important emerging delivery technique in human medicine, with many useful applications for future use in exotic mammal medicine.

As rabbits and rodents are living longer in captivity, veterinarians are encountering geriatric diseases that have not been considered common presentations. Chronic disease conditions such as chronic renal failure require the administration of long-term administration of subcutaneous (SC) fluids. The GIF tube implant kit (GIF-Tube; PractiVet, Phoenix, AZ, USA) is a silicone catheter designed for long-term implantation in the subcutis for administration of fluids. Though designed for dogs and cats, there is a recent report of the use of the GIF tube implant in rabbits with chronic renal failure.[13]

ANTIBACTERIAL AGENTS
Marbofloxacin

Marbofloxacin is a fluoroquinolone antibacterial agent developed exclusively for veterinary use and is currently being studied in exotic mammals. This antibiotic has a wide bactericidal activity spectrum, including primarily gram-negative pathogens, some gram-positive pathogens, and *Mycoplasma* spp. Marbofloxacin was shown to be the most effective agent against bacterial strains isolated from rabbits diagnosed with upper respiratory tract disease when compared with enrofloxacin, danofloxacin, oxytetracycline, or doxycycline.[14] The pharmacokinetics of marbofloxacin have been studied in many species, but few reports are available on its disposition in rabbits.[15–17] Interestingly, the terminal half-life of marbofloxacin was shorter when administered SC compared with either the intramuscular or the intravenous (IV) route,[17] although a very high bioavailability was identified for marbofloxacin when administered through the intramuscular and SC routes.[16,17] Fluoroquinolones exhibit concentration-dependent bactericidal activity. Consequently, the pharmacodynamic ratios C_{max}/minimum inhibitory concentration 90 (MIC90) and AUC24/MIC90 are the best parameters for predicting the antimicrobial effect of fluoroquinolones.[18] Previous investigations have shown that for fluoroquinolones C_{max}/MIC90 greater than 3 produced 99% reduction in bacterial count and C_{max}/MIC90 of 8 or greater prevented the emergence of resistant organisms.[19] In a recent study evaluating the MICs of 27 *Staphylococcus aureus* isolates from a rabbit colony, comparison of previous pharmacokinetic data with MIC data from this study suggested that marbofloxacin at 2 mg/kg would not be effective against these isolates.[17,20] However, oral dosages of 5-mg/kg marbofloxacin administered every 24 hours were determined to be beneficial for susceptible bacteria depending on the MIC value of the targeted pathogen.[15] As marbofloxacin has activity against a wide range of gram-positive and gram-negative bacteria, this antimicrobial agent should be useful against many infections of the skin, urinary tract, and soft tissues. To the author's knowledge, marbofloxacin has not been evaluated in any other exotic mammal species to date.

ANTIFUNGAL AGENTS
Terbinafine

Terbinafine is a synthetic allylamine antifungal medication used commonly in human and veterinary medicine. It inhibits squalene epoxidase, a key enzyme in ergosterol biosynthesis,[21] thereby decreasing ergosterol synthesis and causing toxic levels of squalene to accumulate in the fungal cell. Owing to its mechanisms of action, terbinafine has both fungistatic and fungicidal properties. Terbinafine has been scientifically investigated in the laboratory in several species of exotic mammals. Terbinafine given at a dose of 160 mg/kg orally once a day controlled *Pneumocystis carinii* infection in a rat pneumonia model.[22] Terbinafine alone or in combination at daily oral doses between 150 and 250 mg/kg was effective in treating chromoblastomycosis and *Fusarium verticillioides* in mice.[23,24] However, in rabbits experimentally infected with coccidiomycosis and aspergillosis, terbinafine dosed at 100 or 200 mg/kg orally, every 24 hours had no significant effect on disease progression.[25,26]

Voriconazole

Voriconazole is a new triazole antifungal agent with potent, wide-spectrum activity. The pharmacokinetic activity and metabolism of voriconazole have been studied in the mouse, rat, rabbit, and guinea pig after single and multiple administrations by both oral and IV routes.[27] Oral absorption of voriconazole was essentially complete in all species and pharmacokinetic parameters were dose dependent. Following multiple administrations, autoinduction of metabolism was observed in the mouse and rat, but not in the guinea pig or rabbit. This suggests that plasma concentrations may not remain at a steady state with multiple dosing in the species with autoinduction, thereby creating the need for higher dosages, more frequent dosing, or alternative choices for antifungal therapy.[27] The pharmacokinetic activity and efficacy of oral voriconazole were evaluated in a dermatophytosis guinea pig model.[28] Guinea pigs inoculated with *Microsporum canis* conidia were administered voriconazole at 20 mg/kg orally every 24 hours for 12 days. Skin scrapings from 7 of 8 animals in the voriconazole-treated group had no positive findings on microscopy and culture studies at day 14. Orally administered voriconazole also led to skin concentrations greater than the necessary MICs for *Microsporum* spp; however, to date, activity against other dermatophytes has not been evaluated. Topical administration of 1% voriconazole achieved MICs in the aqueous and vitreous humors of rabbits for organisms most commonly involved in human fungal endophthalmitis, but currently, frequent dosing (every 2 hours) limits the use of this route of administration in rabbits.[29]

ANTIPARASITIC AGENTS
Ivermectin

The efficacy of ivermectin-compounded feed (approximate ingested dose 1.3 mg/kg) for 1, 4, or 8 consecutive weeks was evaluated in vivaria holding approximately 30,000 cages of C57BL/6NCrl mice infested with *Myobia musculi* and *Myocoptes musculinus*. Regardless of treatment duration, all treated mice and contact sentinels remained free of these ectoparasites for as long as 21 weeks after treatment. No adverse side effects associated with ivermectin use were observed in the treated mice. Subsequently, facility-wide treatment was implemented in an attempt to eradicate fur mites from 3 vivaria housing approximately 120,000 mice. Medicated feed was provided for 8 weeks to ensure that all cages and mice were treated. Approximately 14,500 skin scrape samples were evaluated during the 12-months posttreatment surveillance period. All samples were negative for the presence of mites.[30]

Selamectin

Many studies have been recently published evaluating the efficacy of selamectin in exotic mammals. In rabbits, selamectin at 20 mg/kg was rapidly absorbed transdermally but was also rapidly eliminated, suggesting that topical administration of 20 mg/kg every 7 days may be necessary for efficacious treatment of flea infestation in rabbits.[31] Topical application of selamectin at dosages of 6 to 18 mg/kg has been successful in eliminating *Psoroptes cuniculi, Sarcoptes scabiei*, and *Leporacarus gibbus* mites from naturally infested rabbits.[32–34] A single topical application of selamectin at 12 mg/kg was effective in treating cheyletiellosis in rabbits for up to 5 weeks with no adverse effects.[35] Selamectin applied topically at a single dose of 15 mg/kg eliminated *Trixacarus caviae* mites from guinea pigs within 30 days.[36] A breeding colony of 250 different strains of mice was treated with selamectin at 10 mg/kg for 2 treatments 10 days apart for *M musculinus*.[37] Although no apparent ill effects were noted, egg casings were still identified on cellophane tape preparations for up to 6 months after treatment, prompting concern about the effectiveness of selamectin in treating mouse mites. Moxidectin was more effective in eradicating the mites, with negative results on cellophane tape examinations for 2 to 12 months after treatment.[37] Selamectin has been reported to be effective against the ear mite *Otodectes cynotis* when used topically at 6 mg/kg given 28 days apart in ferrets.[38]

Toltrazuril

Toltrazuril, a broad-spectrum anticoccidial drug, is effective against both schizont and gamont stages of *Eimeria* spp.[39] Toltrazuril is very well absorbed through the gastrointestinal tract and rapidly metabolized in rabbits after oral administration.[40] A single oral dose of either 2.5- or 5-mg/kg toltrazuril significantly reduced fecal oocyst counts of several intestinal *Eimeria* spp in rabbits.[41] Treatment with toltrazuril was also highly effective in reducing fecal oocyst output of *Eimeria steidae* in experimentally infected rabbits, and necropsy of these animals showed no significant lesions related to hepatic coccidiosis.[42]

ANALGESIC AGENTS

Multimodal analgesia has become part of our analgesic "best practices" in exotic mammal medicine. The process of nociception and pain involves many steps and pathways, so a single analgesic agent is unlikely to completely alleviate pain in the exotic animal patient. Multimodal analgesic treatment regimens include drugs of different classes that act at differing parts of the pain pathways. For example, patients can be premedicated with an opioid medication and a tranquilizer to modulate pain and stress, ketamine used as a part of the induction protocol can reduce excitement, local anesthetic blocks can be added to inhibit pain transmission, and nonsteroidal anti-inflammatory drugs can be added preoperatively or postoperatively to reduce inflammation and pain. This approach allows smaller dosages of each drug to be used as analgesic effects can be synergistic in activity and may reduce undesirable adverse effects from larger dosages of individual drugs.

Regional infiltration of incision lines and specific peripheral nerve blocks (eg, brachial plexus and sciatic) as well as dental nerve blocks are very useful in multimodal analgesic therapeutic protocols. Intratesticular blocks can be used during castration; the author uses 1 mg/kg of 2% lidocaine per testicle. The toxic dose of local anesthetics in exotic mammals appears to be similar to that observed in cats and dogs. Toxicity is prevented by using appropriate concentrations and volumes of analgesic agents. New long-acting local anesthetic formulations have been shown to produce nerve blocks for 5 days without toxic effects in rats.[43] Eutectic mixture of local anesthetics is a mixture of 2.5% lidocaine and 2.5% prilocaine used topically to desensitize the skin for catheter placement or superficial biopsies. Reported optimal contact time requires application and occlusion with a bandage for 30 to 60 minutes. Eutectic mixture of local anesthetics toxicity is associated with application to large or traumatized areas and prolonged contact time. Systemic uptake may occur in smaller patients if the skin is damaged during shaving.

Epidural anesthesia/analgesia can be an extremely useful adjunct to a multimodal anesthesia/analgesia protocol and can significantly reduce the concentration of inhalant anesthetics for surgical procedures (**Table 1**). Anesthetic/analgesic effects are achieved with little to no systemic drug effects, further reducing the use of other cardiopulmonary depressant anesthetics in the protocol. Epidural anesthesia is more commonly used in larger exotic mammals[44,45] but can be performed routinely in smaller species as well.[46,47] The lumbosacral junction site is the most common site for application of the epidural anesthetic agent(s), and the administration techniques are similar to those used for dogs and cats. Morphine is commonly used at this site because it has a high potency and long duration of analgesic action (18–24 hours), but oxymorphone and buprenorphine have similar effects and duration (see **Table 1**). Bupivacaine at concentrations 0.125% or less appears to have the least motor effect while producing a good sensory block, which is important for minimizing recovery stress and potential patient trauma (see **Table 1**). There appears to be synergism in the epidural space between local analgesics and opioids; drug combinations reduce doses and minimize potential adverse effects of each drug. In general, the total epidural administration volume for all drugs combined should be 0.33 mL/kg or less.

Constant rate infusions (CRIs) are delivered IV at a constant rate over a period of time. CRIs allow the drug to be titrated to effect, which can result in reductions in the total volume of drug used, fewer adverse effects, more consistent analgesia, and reduced cost. A disadvantage with this technique is a slow rise in plasma concentrations to therapeutic concentrations; therefore, a loading dose of the drug is usually administered before initiating the CRI. CRIs should be administered using a syringe pump system owing to the small volumes necessary, even in rabbit and ferret patients. Microdoses of ketamine via IV CRI can be an effective analgesic (**Table 2**). Ketamine is very useful in patients that cannot be intubated, as it has low potential for respiratory

Table 1
Injectable drugs used for epidural anesthesia/analgesia in small exotic mammals

Injectable Epidural Drugs	Rabbit	Ferret	Guinea Pig	Chinchilla	Rat	Mouse	Comments
Buprenorphine (μg/kg)	12	12	12	12	12	—	—
Bupivacaine (0.125%) (mg/kg)	1	1	1	1	1	1	Concentrations of 0.125% or less minimize motor blockade
Morphine (mg/kg)	0.1	0.1	0.1	0.1	0.1	0.1	Little evidence of systemic uptake

These are suggested dosages based on published information and the author's clinical experience. Species and individual variation in response to a drug or combination of drugs may be uncertain, and doses should be adjusted for the needs of each patient. All drugs should be diluted with preservative-free saline only. Total volumes for epidural administration should not exceed 0.33 mL/kg, regardless of drug or drug combination. Opioid and local anesthetics can be administered in combination to reduce the dosage needed of each drug. Use preservative-free formulations for epidural administration.

Table 2
Injectable drugs administered as constant rate infusions used for perioperative and postoperative analgesia in small exotic mammals

Injectable Analgesics	Rabbit	Ferret	Guinea Pig	Chinchilla	Rat	Mouse	Comments
Butorphanol	Loading dose, 0.2–0.4 mg/kg; maintenance, 0.2–0.4 mg/kg/h	Loading dose, 0.05–0.2 mg/kg; maintenance, 0.1–0.4 mg/kg/h	Loading dose, 0.2–0.4 mg/kg; maintenance, 0.2–0.4 mg/kg/h	Loading dose, 0.2–0.4 mg/kg; maintenance, 0.2–0.4 mg/kg/h	Loading dose, 0.2–0.4 mg/kg; maintenance, 0.2–0.4 mg/kg/h	—	Less respiratory depression than with fentanyl
Fentanyl citrate							
Perioperative CRI	Loading dose, 5–10 µg/kg IV; maintenance, 10–30 µg/kg/h IV	Loading dose, 5–10 µg/kg IV; maintenance, 10–30 µg/kg/h IV	Loading dose, 5–10 µg/kg IV; maintenance, 10–30 µg/kg/h IV	Loading dose, 5–10 µg/kg IV; maintenance, 10–30 µg/kg/h IV	—	1.25 mg/kg/h IV	The authors have commonly used up to 60 µg/kg/h in rabbits; apnea common, expect to ventilate patient; Combine with ketamine CRI to reduce overall doses
Postoperative analgesia	1.25–5.0 µg/kg/h	1.25–5.0 µg/kg/h	1.25–5.0 µg/kg/h	1.25–5.0 µg/kg/h	—	—	
Ketamine							
Perioperative CRI	Loading dose, 2–5 mg/kg IV; maintenance, 0.3–1.2 mg/kg/h IV	Loading dose, 2–5 mg/kg IV; maintenance, 0.3–1.2 mg/kg/h IV	Loading dose, 2–5 mg/kg IV; maintenance, 0.3–1.2 mg/kg/h IV	Loading dose, 2–5 mg/kg IV; maintenance, 0.3–1.2 mg/kg/h IV	—	—	More useful when intubation is not possible because less respiratory depression than opioids given CRI; Can be combined with fentanyl to reduce overall doses of both drugs
Postoperative analgesia	0.1–0.4 mg/kg/h	0.1–0.4 mg/kg/h	0.1–0.4 mg/kg/h	0.1–0.4 mg/kg/h	0.1–0.4 mg/kg/h	—	

These are suggested dosages based on published information and the author's clinical experience. If using for postoperative analgesia only, a loading dose should also be used. Gradually wean from postoperative CRI over 12 to 24 h. Species and individual variation in response to a drug or combination of drugs can be uncertain, so the dosage should be adjusted depending on the clinical response of the animal.

depression at CRI doses. Opioid medications can also be used through CRI infusion. All μ receptor agonists can cause respiratory depression, and thus they should be used only when an airway is secure and ventilation is available.[48]

Acupuncture has recently become more popular and accepted in veterinary medicine because of the increase in scientifically based studies investigating its mechanism of action and documented results. The main mechanism of action for analgesia using acupuncture techniques appears to be an increased release of endogenous opioids, and the analgesic effects of acupuncture are reversible with naloxone. Many of these studies have been performed in rodents.[49–52] This analgesic modality is proving very beneficial in chronic pain conditions such as osteoarthritis in effected rabbits and rodents.[53]

Morphine, Hydromorphone, and Oxymorphone

Morphine, hydromorphone, and oxymorphone are μ receptor agonists with similar durations of action. Both hydromorphone and oxymorphone have been used by the author in ferrets, rabbits, and some rodents as primary analgesic agents for treatment of moderate to severe pain, and they are also useful for preemptive analgesia and postoperative pain. In ferrets, these drugs cause profound sedation, making assessment of analgesia difficult.[54] Morphine can cause significant histamine release if given IV, whereas neither hydromorphone nor oxymorphone are likely to do this.

Recently, a long-acting liposome-encapsulated hydromorphone (LE-hydromorphone) has been evaluated in rats and dogs.[55–57] When LE-hydromorphone was given preemptively in a rat model of neuropathic pain, it prevented hyperalgesia for 5 days after surgery.[58] LE-hydromorphone prolonged epidural analgesia for arthritis for as long as 96 hours in rats compared with the standard formulation of hydromorphone, but adverse central nervous system side effects were identified, which warrants careful consideration before use.[56]

Fentanyl/Remifentanil

Fentanyl citrate has an effect for only approximately 30 minutes after a single IV injection, and is thus most commonly used as a CRI during the perianesthetic and postoperative periods.[48] As with all μ receptor agonists, fentanyl can cause respiratory depression, and thus a secure airway and ability to ventilate are required when using it as a CRI. Systemic uptake of transdermal fentanyl in rabbits with a 25-μg/h patch was highest with the longest duration of activity (3 days) when the hair was clipped at the patch site, but the rabbits were more sedated and had a shorter duration of plasma concentrations when the hair was chemically depilated, and no systemic concentrations were identified when hair was present at the patch site.[59] Although extrapolated effective therapeutic plasma concentrations were obtained, loss of body weight occurred in this study. If fentanyl is used for analgesia in rabbits and rodents, appetite and fecal output must be carefully monitored during use.

Remifentanil is an ultrashort-acting μ agonist opioid, making it very suitable for CRI.[48,49,60] Remifentanil is metabolized by esterase hydrolysis in the blood and tissues, not via the liver or kidneys, and thus accumulation is prevented even when administered at high doses over prolonged periods. As remifentanil has a very short half-life, undesirable respiratory and cardiovascular effects are not expected to last for more than 10 to 15 minutes after discontinuation. Acute tolerance can develop with remifentanil,[60,61] which may require increasing doses to maintain intraoperative analgesia. Butorphanol has also been used successfully as a CRI in the clinical setting, but there are no published data for small exotic mammals.

Buprenorphine

Buprenorphine is the preferred analgesic opioid medication used in exotic mammals for postoperative treatment for mild to moderate pain because of its longer duration of effect.[62] Tolerance to buprenorphine after multiple dosing has recently been reported. Rats dosed with buprenorphine at 0.1 mg/kg twice a day for 10 days demonstrated tolerance to antinociception by day 8.[63] Buprenorphine is considered safe and effective when administered at 0.01 to 0.05-mg/kg parenterally, but higher doses are occasionally necessary in smaller mammals. For example, 0.5 mg/kg was safely administered every 6 to 8 hours for analgesia in rats, while 2 mg/kg given every 3 to 5 hours was also found to be safe for mice.[64] In another study, 0.05-mg/kg buprenorphine was sufficient to provide rats postoperative analgesia when given every 12 hours for up to 60 hours.[65] Thus, it is possible that different strains of small mammals might respond differently to different doses of this drug. Buprenorphine administered orally in gelatin to rats was effective at 8 to 10 times the parenteral dose.[66] Oral transmucosal buprenorphine is used in cats, and anecdotally in ferrets, but no studies have been performed to evaluate analgesic efficacy using this route of drug delivery in any exotic mammal species to date. Transdermal buprenorphine has recently been developed for use in human patients.[67] A transdermal hydrogel buprenorphine patch providing one-fifth of the human dose was found to provide human analgesic plasma concentrations in rabbits for 72 hours and was also found to be safe after multiple applications.[68] Although this patch is not yet commercially available, this new route of administration may be useful for longer durations of administration in the future for exotic mammal patients.

Recently, reports of the use of sustained-release buprenorphine (BUP-SR) have been published.[69] Rats administered 1.2 mg/kg SC of sustained-release formulation showed antinociception for 48 to 72 hours.[69] The documented duration of action of standard buprenorphine HCl is as short as 3 to 5 hours in mice, but a recent study evaluating BUP-SR in young adult male BALB/cJ and SWR/J mice showed the analgesic efficacy of BUP-SR appeared to last at least 12 hours.[70] Taken together, these results indicate that this formulation of buprenorphine may be a viable future option for increasing the duration of postsurgical analgesia in exotic mammals.

Meloxicam

Meloxicam has become the most widely used nonsteroidal anti-inflammatory drug in pet exotic animal practice. Some research investigations suggest that some rodents and rabbits need higher meloxicam doses than dogs, but clinical efficacy and safety studies are necessary to determine appropriate meloxicam analgesic doses and dosing frequencies in exotic mammal patients.[71] A recent study evaluating the pharmacokinetics of single or repeated oral doses (daily for 5 days) of 1 mg/kg of meloxicam in 8-month-old rabbits showed that maximal plasma concentrations were much higher than in previous studies in rabbits using lower dosages.[72–74] Clinical efficacy was not evaluated in this study, but meloxicam plasma concentrations were similar to those associated with clinical efficacy in other species at this dose.[74] Transdermal delivery of 0.3% meloxicam in various delivery vehicles has recently been reported in rabbits, suggesting that this route of administration can deliver therapeutically relevant amounts of meloxicam in vivo.[75]

Tramadol

Tramadol hydrochloride is an analgesic agent that has become very popular despite relatively minimal evidence as to its appropriate dosing and efficacy in small mammals. Tramadol is active at opiate, α-adrenergic, and serotonergic receptors.[76] Tramadol is a very weak μ-agonist opioid, whereas the O-desmethyl metabolite (M1) is a much more potent agonist. The conversion to the M1 metabolite is variable among species, but it is known that it is produced in rats, mice, and rabbits.[77–79] In the United States, only the oral formulation is available. In humans, less respiratory depression and constipation are seen with tramadol than with other μ-agonist opioids. The pharmacokinetics of tramadol have been evaluated in rats[78,80,81] and rabbits,[77] but analgesic plasma concentrations have not yet been established in these species. Clinically insignificant isoflurane-sparing effects have been shown in both rats and rabbits administered 10 and 4.4 mg/kg of tramadol orally, respectively,[82,83] and 10-mg/kg doses of oral tramadol did not provide sufficient analgesia to rats after a surgical incision.[65] Significant decreases in heart rate and transient decreases in systolic arterial pressure were identified in rabbits after a single 4.4-mg/kg IV dose.[82] Results of several studies in rats have shown that tramadol can be an effective analgesic for acute pain.[84–87] In rats, tramadol provided analgesia for osteoarthritis,[84] but its efficacy decreased with increased duration of pain, and its antinociceptive mechanism changed over time, which may partially explain its inconsistent efficacy in patients with chronic pain.[85] Anecdotally, oral tramadol doses of 2 to 10 mg/kg have been well tolerated in rabbits and rats. In 1 study, there was evidence of tolerance in rats with chronic use; therefore, dosing may need to be readjusted based on individual needs.[88] Tramadol administered perineurally at a dose of 5 mg/kg was found to be as effective as 2% lidocaine for use for sciatic nerve block in male Wistar rats.[89] Although this analgesic holds great promise for use in exotic mammals, much work is still needed to evaluate appropriate dosing, efficacy, and safety of this drug in different exotic mammal species.

OTHER DRUGS
Deslorelin Acetate

One of the most important new nonantimicrobial, nonanesthetic/analgesic medications available is deslorelin acetate (Suprelorin F; Virbac Animal Health, Fort Worth, TX, USA). Deslorelin acetate is a synthetic analogue of gonadorelin and is legally marketed as a Food and Drug Administration-indexed product for ferrets only in the United States for adrenocortical disease (ACD). Deslorelin acetate is formulated in an SC, controlled-release implant. Like other gonadotropin-releasing hormone analogues, deslorelin acetate stimulates luteinizing hormone and follicle-stimulating hormone secretion, which desensitizes the pituitary gland by downregulating gonadotropin-releasing hormone receptors, which in turn effectively decreases release of gonadotropins. Ferrets receiving a single 4.7-mg slow-release implant had improvement in clinical signs of ACD within 2 weeks, and plasma hormone concentrations remained decreased until recurrence of clinical signs was noted 8.5 to 20.5 months later (mean = 13.7 months).[90] Pretreatment and posttreatment concentrations of estradiol, rostenedione, and 17-OH progesterone were significantly different in ferrets studied.[90] The time from treatment to return of ACD signs was longer for ferrets implanted with deslorelin (16.5 months) compared with the surgery group (13.6 months).[91] A single implant appears to have a significant increase in duration of effect over leuprolide acetate treatment; however, similarly to leuprolide acetate, it does not seem to deter tumor growth or metastasis.[92] Although currently only labeled for ferrets in the United States for ACD, the 4.7-mg implant has also been evaluated to assess contraceptive efficacy. Plasma follicle-stimulating hormone and testosterone concentrations, size of testicles, and spermatogenesis were all suppressed after the use of a deslorelin implant in male ferrets.[93] Fecal progesterone concentrations were decreased in female ferrets for 698 days following deslorelin acetate treatment; however, only 60% of treated ferrets returned to fertility by the second posttreatment mating.[94] In female rats, changes in vaginal cytology occurred at 2 weeks following implantation, and none of the rats conceived during the 4 months of the experiment. Additionally, 38 pet rats were recruited from clients in practice to test for potential adverse effects, including 6 males and 32 females with a mean age of 14 months. According to this pilot study, deslorelin implants might also be useful as a contraceptive method in female rats.[95] The 4.7-mg deslorelin acetate implant used in guinea pigs with cystic ovaries did not significantly reduce the size of the ovarian cysts during the treatment.[96] This would be expected as most ovarian cysts in guinea pigs are serous cysts (cystic rete ovarii), and thus would not be hormone responsive.[97]

REFERENCES

1. Küster T, Zumkehr B, Hermann C, et al. Voluntary ingestion of antiparasitic drugs emulsified in honey represents an alternative to gavage in mice. J Am Assoc Lab Anim Sci 2012;51:219–23.
2. Aiken S. Surgical treatment of dental abscesses in rabbits. In: Quesenberry KE, Carpenter JW, editors. Ferrets, rabbits, and rodents: clinical medicine and surgery. 2nd edition. Philadelphia: WB Saunders Co; 2004. p. 379–82.
3. Bennett RA. Management of abscesses of the head in rabbits. Proceedings of the 13th North American Veterinary Conference; Orlando, 1999. p. 821–3.
4. Hernandez-Divers SJ. Mandibular abscess treatment using antibiotic impregnated beads. Exotic DVM 2000;2:5–18.
5. Hernandez-Divers SJ. Molar disease and abscesses in rabbits. Exotic DVM 2001; 3:64–9.
6. Taylor WM, Beaufrere H, Mans C, et al. Long-term outcome of treatment of dental abscesses with a wound- packing technique in pet rabbits: 13 cases (1998-2007). J Am Vet Med Assoc 2010;237:1444–9.
7. Ward ML. Diagnosis and management of a retrobulbar abscess of periapical origin in a domestic rabbit. Vet Clin North Am Exot Anim Pract 2006;9:657–65.
8. Harcourt-Brown FM. Abscesses. In: Harcourt-Brown FM, editor. Textbook of rabbit medicine. Oxford (England): Butterworth Heinemann, Elsevier Science; 2002. p. 206–23.
9. Remeeus PG, Verbeek M. The use of calcium hydroxide in the treatment of abscesses in the cheek of the rabbit resulting from a dental periapical disorder. J Vet Dent 1995;12:19–22.
10. Harcourt-Brown FM. Treatment of facial abscesses in rabbits. Exotic DVM 1999;1: 83–8.
11. Seliktar D. Designing cell-compatible hydrogels for biomedical applications. Science 2012;336:1124–8.
12. Marchesan S, Qu Y, Waddington LJ, et al. Self-assembly of ciprofloxacin and a tripeptide into an antimicrobial nano- structured hydrogel. Biomaterials 2013; 34:3678–87.
13. Lennox AM. Care of the geriatric rabbit. Vet Clin North Am Exot Anim Pract 2010; 13:123–33.
14. Rougier S, Galland D, Boucher S, et al. Epidemiology and susceptibility of pathogenic bacteria responsible for upper respiratory tract infections in pet rabbits. Vet Microbiol 2006;115:192–8.

15. Carpenter JW, Pollock CG, Koch DE, et al. Single- and multiple-dose pharmaco-kinetics of marbofloxacin after oral administration to rabbits. Am J Vet Res 2009; 70:522–6.

16. Abo-El-Sooud K, Goudah A. Influence of Pasteurella multocida infection on the pharmacokinetic behavior of marbofloxacin after intravenous and intramuscular administrations in rabbits. J Vet Pharmacol Ther 2009;33:63–8.

17. Marín P, Álamo LF, Escudero E, et al. Pharmacokinetics of marbofloxacin in rabbits after intravenous, intramuscular, and subcutaneous administration. Res Vet Sci 2013;94:698–700.

18. Lode H, Borner K, Koeppe P. Pharmacodynamics of fluoroquinolones. Clin Infect Dis 1998;27:33–9.

19. Craig WA. Pharmacokinetic/pharmacodynamic parameters: rationale for antibac-terial dosing of mice and men. Clin Infect Dis 1998;26:1–10.

20. Marín P, Álamo L, Escudero E, et al. Fluoroquinolone susceptibility of Staphylo-coccus aureus strains isolated from commercial rabbit farms in Spain. Vet Rec 2012;170:519–20.

21. Nowosielski M, Hoffman M, Wyrwicz LS, et al. Detailed mechanism of squalene epoxidase inhibition by terbinafine. J Chem Inf Model 2011;51:455–62.

22. Artan MO, Koç N, Öztürk A. Evaluation of terbinafine activity on Pneumocystis carinii in the rat model. Trakya Univ Tip Fak Derg 2010;27:331–3.

23. Calvo E, Pastor FJ, Mayayo E, et al. Antifungal therapy in an athymic murine model of chromoblastomycosis by Fonsecaea pedrosoi. Antimicrob Agents Chemother 2011;55:3709–13.

24. Ruíz-Cendoya M, Pastor FJ, Capilla J, et al. Treatment of murine Fusarium verti-cillioides infection with liposomal amphotericin B plus terbinafine. Int J Antimicrob Agents 2011;37:58–61.

25. Sorensen KN, Sobel RA, Clemons KV, et al. Comparative efficacies of terbinafine and fluconazole in treatment of experimental coccidioidal meningitis in a rabbit model. Antimicrob Agents Chemother 2000;44:3087–91.

26. Kirkpatrick WR, Vallor AC, McAtee RK, et al. Combination therapy with terbinafine and amphotericin B in a rabbit model of experimental invasive aspergillosis. Antimicrob Agents Chemother 2005;49:4751–3.

27. Roffey SJ, Cole S, Comby P, et al. The disposition of voriconazole in mouse, rat, rabbit, guinea pig, dog, and human. Drug Metab Dispos 2003;31:731–41.

28. Saunte DM, Simmel F, Frimodt-Moller N, et al. In vivo efficacy and pharmacoki-netics of voriconazole in an animal model of dermatophytosis. Antimicrob Agents Chemother 2007;51:3317–21.

29. Wei LC, Tsai TC, Tsai HY, et al. Comparison of voriconazole concentration in the aqueous humor and vitreous between non-scraped and scraped corneal epithelium groups after topical 1% voriconazole application. Curr Eye Res 2010;35:573–9.

30. Arbona RJ, Lipman NS, Wolf FR. Treatment and eradication of murine fur mites: III. Treatment of a large mouse colony with ivermectin-compounded feed. J Am Assoc Lab Anim Sci 2010;49:633–7.

31. Carpenter JW, Dryden MW, Kukanich B. Pharmacokinetics, efficacy, and adverse effects of selamectin following topical administration in flea-infested rabbits. Am J Vet Res 2012;73:562–6.

32. McTier TL, Hair AJ, Walstrom DJ, et al. Efficacy and safety of topical administra-tion of selamectin for treatment of ear mite infestation in rabbits. J Am Vet Med Assoc 2003;223:322–4.

33. Kurtdede A, Karaer Z, Acar A, et al. Use of selamectin for the treatment of psor-optic and sarcoptic mite infestation in rabbits. Vet Dermatol 2007;18:18–22.

34. Birke LL, Molina PE, Baker DG, et al. Comparison of selamectin and imidacloprid plus permethrin in eliminating Leporacarus gibbus infestation in laboratory rabbits (Oryctolagus cuniculus). J Am Assoc Lab Anim Sci 2009;48:757–62.
35. Kim SH, Lee JY, Jun HK, et al. Efficacy of selamectin in the treatment of cheyletiellosis in pet rabbits. Vet Dermatol 2008;19:26–7.
36. Eshar D, Bdolah-Abram T. Comparison of efficacy, safety, and convenience of selamectin versus ivermectin for treatment of Trixacarus caviae mange in pet guinea pigs (Cavia porcellus). J Am Vet Med Assoc 2012;241:1056–8.
37. Mook DM, Benjamin KA. Use of selamectin and moxidectin in the treatment of mouse fur mites. J Am Assoc Lab Anim Sci 2008;47:20–4.
38. Orcutt C, Tater K. Dermatologic diseases. In: Quesenberry KE, Carpenter JW, editors. Ferrets, rabbits, and rodents: clinical medicine and surgery. Philadelphia: Elsevier/Saunders; 2012. p. 122–31.
39. Hu L, Liu C, Shang C, et al. Pharmacokinetics and improved bioavailability of toltrazuril after oral administration to rabbits. J Vet Pharmacol Ther 2010;33: 503–6.
40. Kim MS, Lim JH, Hwang YH, et al. Plasma disposition of toltrazuril and its metabolites, toltrazuril sulfoxide and toltrazuril sulfone, in rabbits after oral administration. Vet Parasitol 2010;169:1–2.
41. Redrobe SP, Gakos G, Elliot SC, et al. Comparison of toltrazuril and sulphadimethoxine in the treatment of intestinal coccidiosis in pet rabbits. Vet Rec 2010;167: 287–90.
42. Cam Y, Atasever A, Eraslan G, et al. Eimeria stiedae: experimental infection in rabbits and the effect of treatment with toltrazuril and ivermectin. Exp Parasitol 2008;19:164–72.
43. Wang CF, Djalali AG, Gandhi A, et al. An absorbable local anesthetic matrix provides several days of functional sciatic nerve blockade. Anesth Analg 2009; 108:1027–33.
44. Hughes PJ, Doherty MM, Charman WN. A rabbit model for the evaluation of epidurally administered local anaesthetic agents. Anaesth Intensive Care 1993; 21:298–303.
45. Dollo G, Malinovsky JM, Peron A, et al. Prolongation of epidural bupivacaine effects with hyaluronic acid in rabbits. Int J Pharm 2004;272:109–19.
46. Morimoto K, Nishimura R, Matsunaga S, et al. Epidural analgesia with a combination of bupivacaine and buprenorphine in rats. J Vet Med A Physiol Pathol Clin Med 2001;48:303–12.
47. Eisele PH, Kaaekuahiwi MA, Canfield DR, et al. Epidural catheter placement for testing of obstetrical analgesics in female guinea pigs. Lab Anim Sci 1994;44: 486–90.
48. Criado AB, Gomez de Segura IA. Reduction of isoflurane MAC by fentanyl or remifentanil in rats. Vet Anaesth Analg 2003;30:250–6.
49. Yang J, Liu WY, Song CY, et al. Through central arginine vasopressin, not oxytocin and endogenous opiate peptides, glutamate sodium induces hypothalamic paraventricular nucleus enhancing acupuncture analgesia in the rat. Neurosci Res 2006;54:49–56.
50. Huang C, Wang Y, Han JS, et al. Characteristics of electroacupuncture-induced analgesia in mice: variation with strain, frequency, intensity and opioid involvement. Brain Res 2002;945:20–5.
51. Koo ST, Park YI, Lim KS, et al. Acupuncture analgesia in a new rat model of ankle sprain pain. Pain 2002;99:423–31.

52. Zhang RX, Lao L, Wang X, et al. Electroacupuncture combined with indomethacin enhances antihyperalgesia in inflammatory rats. Pharmacol Biochem Behav 2004;78:793–7.
53. Koski MA. Acupuncture for zoological companion animals. Vet Clin North Am Exot Anim Pract 2011;14:141–54.
54. Johnston MS. Clinical approaches to analgesia in ferrets and rabbits. J Exot Pet Med 2005;14:229–35.
55. Krugner-Higby L, Smith L, Schmidt B, et al. Experimental pharmacodynamics and analgesic efficacy of liposome- encapsulated hydromorphone in dogs. J Am Anim Hosp Assoc 2011;47:185–95.
56. Schmidt JR, Krugner-Higby L, Heath TD, et al. Epidural administration of liposome-encapsulated hydromorphone provides extended analgesia in a rodent model of stifle arthritis. J Am Assoc Lab Anim Sci 2011;50:507–12.
57. Smith LJ, Kukanich BK, Krugner-Higby LA, et al. Pharmacokinetics of ammonium sulfate gradient loaded liposome-encapsulated oxymorphone and hydromorphone in healthy dogs. Vet Anaesth Analg 2013;40:537–45.
58. Smith LJ, Valenzuela JR, Krugner-Higby LA, et al. A single dose of liposome-encapsulated hydromorphone provides extended analgesia in a rat model of neuropathic pain. Comp Med 2006;56:487–92.
59. Foley PL, Henderson AL, Bissonette EA, et al. Evaluation of fentanyl transdermal patches in rabbits: blood concentrations and physiologic response. Comp Med 2001;51:239–44.
60. Gomez de Segura IA, de la Vibora JB, Aguado D. Opioid tolerance blunts the reduction in the sevoflurane minimum alveolar concentration produced by remifentanil in the rat. Anesthesiology 2009;110:1133–8.
61. Hayashida M, Fukunaga A, Hanaoka K. Detection of acute tolerance to the analgesic and nonanalgesic effects of remifentanil infusion in a rabbit model. Anesth Analg 2003;97:1347–52.
62. Roughan JV, Flecknell PA. Buprenorphine: a reappraisal of its antinociceptive effects and therapeutic use in alleviating post-operative pain in animals. Lab Anim 2002;36:322–43.
63. Wala EP, Holtman JR Jr. Buprenorphine-induced hyperalgesia in the rat. Eur J Pharmacol 2011;651:89–95.
64. Gades NM, Danneman PJ, Wixson SK, et al. The magnitude and duration of the analgesic effect of morphine, butorphanol, and buprenorphine in rats and mice. Contemp Top Lab Anim Sci 2000;39:8–13.
65. McKeon GP, Pacharinsak C, Long CT, et al. Analgesic effects of tramadol, tramadol-gabapentin, and buprenorphine in an incisional model of pain in rats (Rattus norvegicus). J Am Assoc Lab Anim Sci 2011;50:192–7.
66. Flecknell PA. Analgesia of small mammals. Vet Clin North Am Exot Anim Pract 2001;4:47–56.
67. Weiner M, Sarantopoulos C, Gordon E. Transdermal buprenorphine controls central neuropathic pain. J Opioid Manag 2012;8:414–5.
68. Park I, Kim D, Song J, et al. Buprederm, a new transdermal delivery system of buprenorphine: pharmacokinetic, efficacy and skin irritancy studies. Pharm Res 2008;25:1052–62.
69. Foley PL, Liang H, Crichlow AR. Evaluation of a sustained-release formulation of buprenorphine for analgesia in rats. J Am Assoc Lab Anim Sci 2011;50:198–204.
70. Carbone ET, Lindstrom KE, Diep S, et al. Duration of action of sustained-release buprenorphine in 2 strains of mice. J Am Assoc Lab Anim Sci 2012;51:815–9.

71. Roughan JV, Flecknell PA. Evaluation of a short duration behaviour-based post-operative pain scoring system in rats. Eur J Pain 2003;7:397–406.
72. Turner PV, Chen HC, Taylor WM. Pharmacokinetics of meloxicam in rabbits after single and repeat oral dosing. Comp Med 2006;56:63–7.
73. Carpenter JW, Pollock CG, Koch DE, et al. Single and multiple-dose pharmaco-kinetics of meloxicam after oral administration to the rabbit (Oryctolagus cuniculus). J Zoo Wildl Med 2009;40:601–6.
74. Fredholm DV, Carpenter JW, Kukanich B, et al. Pharmacokinetics of meloxicam in rabbits after oral administration of single and multiple doses. Am J Vet Res 2013; 74:636–41.
75. Patel M, Joshi A, Hassanzadeth H, et al. Quantification of dermal and transdermal delivery of meloxicam gels in rabbits. Drug Dev Ind Pharm 2011;37:613–7.
76. Scott LJ, Perry CM. Tramadol: a review of its use in perioperative pain. Drugs 2000;60:139–76.
77. Souza MJ, Greenacre CB, Cox SK. Pharmacokinetics of orally administered tra-madol in domestic rabbits (Oryctolagus cuniculus). Am J Vet Res 2008;69: 979–82.
78. Parasrampuria R, Vuppugalla R, Elliott K, et al. Route- dependent stereoselective pharmacokinetics of tramadol and its active O-demethylated metabolite in rats. Chirality 2007;19:190–6.
79. Wu WN, McKown LA, Codd EE, et al. Metabolism of two analgesic agents, tramadol-n-oxide and tramadol, in specific pathogen-free and axenic mice. Xenobiotica 2006;36:551–65.
80. Garrido MJ, Sayar O, Segura C, et al. Pharmacokinetic/pharmacodynamic modeling of the antinociceptive effects of (+)-tramadol in the rat: role of cyto-chrome P450 2D activity. J Pharmacol Exp Ther 2003;305:710–8.
81. Zhao Y, Tao T, Wu J, et al. Pharmacokinetics of tramadol in rat plasma and cere-brospinal fluid after intranasal administration. J Pharm Pharmacol 2008;60: 1149–54.
82. Egger CM, Souza MJ, Greenacre CB, et al. Effect of intravenous administration of tramadol hydrochloride on the minimum alveolar concentration of isoflurane in rabbits. Am J Vet Res 2009;70:945–9.
83. de Wolff MH, Leather HA, Wouters PF. Effects of tramadol on minimum alveolar concentration (MAC) of isoflurane in rats. Br J Anaesth 1999;83:780–3.
84. Chandran P, Pai M, Blomme EA, et al. Pharmacological modulation of movement-evoked pain in a rat model of osteoarthritis. Eur J Pharmacol 2009;613:39–45.
85. Hama A, Sagen J. Altered antinociceptive efficacy of tramadol over time in rats with painful peripheral neuropathy. Eur J Pharmacol 2007;559:32–7.
86. Guneli E, Karabay Yavasoglu NU, Apaydin S, et al. Analysis of the antinociceptive effect of systemic administration of tramadol and dexmedetomidine combination on rat models of acute and neuropathic pain. Pharmacol Biochem Behav 2007; 88:9–17.
87. Cannon CZ, Kissling GE, Goulding DR, et al. Analgesic effects of tramadol, carprofen or multimodal analgesia in rats undergoing ventral laparotomy. Lab Anim 2011;40:85–93.
88. Valle M, Garrido MJ, Pavon JM, et al. Pharmacokinetic-pharmacodynamic modeling of the antinociceptive effects of main active metabolites of tramadol, (+)-O-desmethyl tramadol and (-)-O-desmethyltramadol, in rats. J Pharmacol Exp Ther 2000;293:646–53.

89. Sousa AM, Ashmawi HA, Costa LS, et al. Percutaneous sciatic nerve block with tramadol induces analgesia and motor blockade in two animal pain models. Braz J Med Biol Res 2012;45:147–52.
90. Wagner RA. The treatment of adrenal cortical disease in ferrets with 4.7-mg deslorelin acetate implants. J Exot Pet Med 2009;18:146–52.
91. Lennox AM, Wagner RA. Comparison of 4.7 mg deslorelin implants and surgery for the treatment of adrenocortical disease in ferrets. J Exot Pet Med 2012;21: 332–5.
92. Wagner RA, Piché CA, Jöchle W, et al. Clinical and endocrine responses to treatment with deslorelin acetate implants in ferrets with adrenocortical disease. Am J Vet Res 2005;66:910–4.
93. Schoemaker NJ, van Deijk R, Muijlaert B, et al. Use of a gonadotropin releasing hormone agonist implant as an alternative for surgical castration in male ferrets (Mustela putorius furo). Theriogen 2008;70:161–7.
94. Prohaczik A, Kulcsar M, Trigg T, et al. Comparison of four treatments to suppress ovarian activity in ferrets (Mustela putorius furo). Vet Rec 2010;166:74–8.
95. Grosset C, Peters S, Peron F, et al. Contraceptive effect and potential side-effects of deslorelin acetate implants in rats (Rattus norvegicus): preliminary observations. Can J Vet Res 2012;76:209–14.
96. Schuetzenhofer G, Goericke-Pesch S, Wehrend A. Effects of deslorelin implants on ovarian cysts in guinea pigs. Schweiz Arch Tierheilkd 2011;153:416–7.
97. Shi F, Petroff BK, Herath CB, et al. Serous cysts are a benign component of the cyclic ovary in the guinea pig with an incidence dependent upon inhibin bioactivity. J Vet Med Sci 2002;64:129–35.

Index

Note: Page numbers of article titles are in **boldface** type.

A

Adrenal gland disease
  in ferrets
    prevention of, 239
Aging
  of ferrets
    illnesses related to
      prevention of, 240
Analgesic agents
  for exotic animals
    advances in, 326–331
      buprenorphine, 330
      described, 326–329
      fentanyl, 329
      hydromorphone, 329
      meloxican, 330
      morphine, 329
      oxymorphone, 329
      remifentanil, 329
      tramadol, 330–331
Antibacterial agents
  for exotic animals
    advances in, 324
Antifungal agents
  for exotic animals
    advances in, 324–325
Antiparasitic agents
  for exotic animals
    advances in, 325–326
Aquatic animals
  environmental enrichment for, **305–321**
    argument for, 305–307
    cephalopods, 318–319
    elasmobranchs, 318
    feeding behavior, 308–309
    filtration, 312–314
    housing, 309–311
    husbandry, 307–312
    koi, 317–318
    life stages–related, 314–317
      display, 315–316
      fish fry, 314

Vet Clin Exot Anim 18 (2015) 339–350
http://dx.doi.org/10.1016/S1094-9194(15)00020-1
1094-9194/15/$ – see front matter © 2015 Elsevier Inc. All rights reserved.

vetexotic.theclinics.com

Aquatic (*continued*)
        quarantine, 314–315
           training for medical procedures, 316–317
     lighting needs, 311–312
     nutrition, 307–308
     species-specific, 317–319
     water quality, 314
Auditory enrichment
  for juvenile psittacines, 227
Autonomy
  for juvenile psittacines, 229–230

B

Behavior(s)
  species-specific
    expression of
      for exotic animals, 192
Behavior training
  for camelids
    for healthy interaction
      with owners, 266–275
  for reptiles
    for healthy interaction
      with conspecifics, 300–301
      with owners, 297–300
Bird(s). *See specific birds, e.g.,* Psittacine(s)
Buprenorphine
  for exotic animals, 330

C

Cage
  for juvenile psittacines, 222
  for small exotic companion mammals, 247–248
Cage substrate
  of psittacine, 201
Camelid(s)
  environmental enrichment for, **262–275**
    behavior training
      for healthy interaction with conspecifics, 277–278
      for healthy interaction with owners, 266–275
    described, 262
    desensitization to human approach, 270–273
    halter fit, 273–275
    handling area setup, 267–270
    mental stimulation, 262–266
  wellness management of, **255–262**
    diet and nutrition, 255–257
    housing and shelter, 257–259
    substrate, 259
    temperature and environment, 259–260

weight-related, 260–262
young
interacting appropriately with, 275–276
Canine distemper virus
in ferrets
prevention of, 237
Car comfort
for juvenile psittacines, 224–225
Cardboard boxes
for small exotic companion mammals, 248
Carrier
for juvenile psittacines, 224–225
Cephalopods
environmental enrichment for, 318–319
Chinchilla(s)
environmental enrichment for, 252
Choice opportunities
for exotic pets, 193–194
Clinical therapeutics
exotic animal
advances in, **323–337**
analgesic agents, 326–331
antibacterial agents, 324
antifungal agents, 324–325
antiparasitic agents, 325–326
deslorelin acetate, 331–332
introduction, 323
therapeutic delivery systems, 323–324
Company
for small exotic companion mammals, 248
Control
opportunities for
for exotic pets, 193–194

D

Deslorelin acetate
for exotic animals, 331–332
Dietary needs
of camelids, 255–257
of exotic pets, 191
Dishes
for juvenile psittacines, 222–223
Display
for aquatic animals, 315–316
Dust baths
for small exotic companion mammals, 250

E

Ectoparasites
in ferrets

Ectoparasites (*continued*)
    prevention of, 237
Elasmobranchs
    environmental enrichment for, 318
Environmental enrichment
    for aquatic animals, **305–321**. *See also* Aquatic animals
    for camelids, **262–275**. *See also* Camelid(s)
    defined, 202, 213
    for ferrets, 241, 242. *See also* Ferret(s)
    for psittacines, **202–208**. *See also* Psittacine(s), environmental
        enrichment for
        juvenile, **213–231**. *See also* Psittacine(s), juvenile, environmental
            enrichment for
    for reptiles, 296–301
    for small exotic companion mammals, **247–253**. *See also* Small exotic
        companion mammals
Exercise
    for psittacines, 205–206
        juvenile, 220–221
Exercise wheels
    for small exotic companion mammals, 248
Exotic animal clinical therapeutics
    advances in, **323–337**. *See also* Clinical therapeutics, exotic animal
Exotic pets
    mental health of, **187–195**. *See also* Mental health, of exotic pets
External home environment
    for juvenile psittacines, 225

F

FECV. *See* Ferret enteric coronavirus (FECV)
Feeders
    for camelids, 258–259
Feeding
    of camelids, 255–259
Feeding behavior
    of aquatic animals, 308–309
Fentanyl
    for exotic animals, 329
Ferret(s), **233–244**
    dietary needs of, 234, 236
    environmental enrichment for, 241, 242, 251
    housing for, 234–236
    husbandry, 234–236
    introduction, 233
    medical wellness management/disease prevention for, 236–240
        infectious disease prevention, 237–238
        noninfectious disease prevention, 238–240
        surgical sterilization, 236
    ownership of
        legal aspects specific to, 233–234

parasitism in
    prevention of, 237
    psychological health management in, 240–243
    training of, 241, 243
    wellness management for, **233–244**
Ferret enteric coronavirus (FECV)
    prevention of, 238
Ferret systemic coronavirus
    prevention of, 238
Filtration
    for aquatic animals, 312–314
Fish fry
    environmental enrichment for, 314
Food hiding
    from small exotic companion mammals, 250
Food recognition
    for juvenile psittacines, 228–229
Foraging
    for psittacines, 205
        juvenile, 229
    for reptiles, 296–297
Foreign bodies
    gastrointestinal
        in ferrets
            prevention of, 238–239

G

Gastritis
    Helicobacter
        in ferrets
            prevention of, 238
Gastrointestinal foreign bodies
    in ferrets
        prevention of, 238–239
Gastrointestinal ulceration
    in ferrets
        prevention of, 239
Geriatric-related illnesses
    in ferrets
        prevention of, 240
Glider(s)
    sugar
        environmental enrichment for, 253
Guinea pigs
    environmental enrichment for, 252

H

Halter fit
    for camelids, 273–275

Hammock(s)
    for small exotic companion mammals, 250–251
Heartworm disease
    in ferrets
        prevention of, 237
Helicobacter gastritis
    in ferrets
        prevention of, 238
Hiding and nesting places
    for small exotic companion mammals, 249
Home environment
    external
        for juvenile psittacines, 225
Housing
    for aquatic animals, 309–311
    for camelids, 257–259
    for psittacines, 200–201
    for reptiles, 287–290
Humidity
    for reptiles, 292–293
Husbandry
    for aquatic animals, 307–312
    of ferrets, 234–236
    of psittacines, 198–201
Hydromorphone
    for exotic animals, 329

I

Influenza
    in ferrets
        prevention of, 238
Insulinoma
    in ferrets
        prevention of, 239
Ivermectin
    for exotic animals, 325

K

Koi
    environmental enrichment for, 317–318

L

Lighting needs
    of aquatic animals, 311–312
    of psittacines, 201
    of reptiles, 294–296
Lymphoma(s)
    in ferrets
        prevention of, 239

M

Marbofloxacin
    for exotic animals, 324
Meloxicam
    for exotic animals, 330
Mental health
    of exotic pets, **187–195**
        domesticated *vs.* wild, 188
        introduction, 187–188
        opportunities to thrive, 190–194
            choice- and control-related, 193–194
            expression of species-specific behavior, 192
            optimal health, 192
            self-maintain, 191–192
            well-balanced diet, 191
        stress and, 188–190
Mental stimulation
    for camelids, 262–266
Morphine
    for exotic animals, 329

N

Nesting places
    for small exotic companion mammals, 249
New World camelids (NWCs), **255–280**. *See also* Camelid(s)
Nutraceuticals
    for reptiles, 286–287
Nutrition
    for aquatic animals, 307–308
    for camelids, 255–256
    for psittacines, 198–200
    for reptiles, 282–287
Nutritional enrichment
    for juvenile psittacines, 228–229
NWCs. *See* New World camelids (NWCs)

O

Occupational enrichment
    for juvenile psittacines, 220–222
        exercise, 220–221
        wing-clipping, 221–222
Optimal health
    for exotic pets, 192
Oxymorphone
    for exotic animals, 329

P

Parasitism
  in ferrets
    prevention of, 237
Perch(es)
  for juvenile psittacines, 223
Physical enrichment
  for juvenile psittacines, 222–225
    cage, 222
    carrier and cars, 224–225
    dishes, 222–223
    external home environment, 225
    perches, 223
    sleep environment, 225
    toys, 224
Prairie dogs
  environmental enrichment for, 253
Psittacine(s)
  environmental enrichment for, **202–208**
    described, 202
    exercise, 205–206
    foraging, 205
    healthy owner and bird interaction in, 207–211
    importance of, 202–203
    introduction, 197–198
    provision of, 203–205
  juvenile
    environmental enrichment for, **213–231**
      autonomy and puberty, 229–230
      introduction, 213–214
      nutritional enrichment, 228–229
      occupational enrichment, 220–222
      physical enrichment, 222–225. *See also* Physical enrichment,
        for juvenile psittacines
      sensory enrichment, 226–228
      social enrichment, 214–220. *See also* Social enrichment, for
        juvenile psittacines
  wellness management of, **197–202**
    cage substrate, 201
    housing, 200–201
    husbandry, 198–201
    introduction, 197–198
    lighting needs, 201
    nutrition, 198–200
    water management, 200
    weight management, 200
Psychological health management
  of ferrets, 240–243
Puberty
  of juvenile psittacines, 229–230

Q

Quarantine
 for aquatic animals, 314–315

R

Rabbit(s)
 environmental enrichment for, 251–252
Rabies
 in ferrets
  prevention of, 237
Remifentanil
 for exotic animals, 329
Reptile(s)
 environmental enrichment for, 296–301
  behavior training
   for healthy interaction with conspecifics, 300–301
   for healthy interaction with owners, 297–300
  described, 296
  foraging, 296–297
  weight management, 297
 wellness management of, **281–304**
  described, 281–282
  housing, 287–290
  lighting, 294–296
  nutrition, 282–286, 286–287
  substrate, 290–292
  temperature, 293–294
  water and humidity, 292–293
Rodent(s)
 environmental enrichment for, 252–253

S

Selamectin
 for exotic animals, 325–326
Self-maintain opportunity
 for exotic pets, 191–192
Sensory enrichment
 for juvenile psittacines, 226–228
  auditory enrichment, 227
  tactile enrichment, 227–228
  visual enrichment, 226
Shelter
 for camelids, 257–259
Sleep environment
 for juvenile psittacines, 225
Small exotic companion mammals. *See also* Guinea pigs; *specific species, e.g.,* Ferret(s)
 environmental enrichment for, **247–253**

Small (*continued*)
    cage, 247–248
    cardboard boxes, 248
    company, 248
    described, 247
    dust baths, 250
    exercise wheels, 248
    food hiding, 250
    general concepts, 247–251
    hammocks, 250–251
    hiding and nesting places, 249
    species-specific ideas, 251–253
    supervised time-out, 248
    toys, 249
    tubes, 249, 250
  introduction, 245–246
  wellness management of, **245–247**
    species-specific veterinary recommendations, 246–247
    veterinary wellness visits, 246
Social enrichment
  for juvenile psittacines, 214–220
    described, 214
    for healthy interaction
      with conspecifics, 215–216
      with nonpreferred or nonowner humans, 218–219
      with owners, 216–218
      with veterinary professionals, 219–220
Species-specific behavior
  expression of
    for exotic animals, 192
Stress
  mental health and, 188–190
Substrate
  for camelids, 259
  of psittacines, 201
  for reptiles, 290–292
Sugar gliders
  environmental enrichment for, 253
Supervised time-out
  for small exotic companion mammals, 248
Surgical sterilization
  for ferrets, 236

T

Tactile enrichment
  for juvenile psittacines, 227–228
Temperature management
  for camelids, 259–260
  for reptiles, 293–294

Terbinafine
    for exotic animals, 324–325
Toltrazuril
    for exotic animals, 326
Toys
    for juvenile psittacines, 224
    for small exotic companion mammals, 249
Tramadol
    for exotic animals, 330–331
Tube(s)
    for small exotic companion mammals, 249, 250

U

Ulceration
    gastrointestinal
        in ferrets
            prevention of, 239
Urolithiasis
    in ferrets
        prevention of, 240

V

Vaccine reactions
    in ferrets
        prevention of, 237–238
Veterinary wellness visits
    for small exotic companion mammals, 246
Viral diseases
    in ferrets
        prevention of, 237–238
Visual enrichment
    for juvenile psittacines, 226
Voriconazole
    for exotic animals, 325

W

Water
    for reptiles, 292–293
Water management
    of psittacines, 200
Water quality
    for aquatic animals, 314
Weight management
    of camelids, 260–262
    of psittacines, 200
    of reptiles, 297
Well-balanced diet

Well-balanced (*continued*)
   for exotic pets, 191
Wellness management
   of camelids, **255–280**. *See also* Camelid(s)
   of ferrets, **233–244**. *See also* Ferret(s)
   of psittacines, **197–201**. *See also* Psittacine(s)
   of reptiles, **281–304**. *See also* Reptile(s)
   of small exotic companion mammals, **245–247**. *See also* Small
      exotic companion mammals
Wing-clipping
   for juvenile psittacines, 221–222

Printed and bound by CPI Group (UK) Ltd, Croydon, CR0 4YY

03/10/2024

01040485-0012